Once Upon A Heart.

Stories from
Le Bonheur Children's Hospital

A heartfelt collection of
60 stories spanning the
hospital's first 60 years.

D0126177

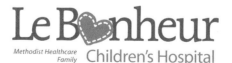

Le B♥nheur
Methodist Healthcare
Family   Children's Hospital

Produced by the Department of Marketing and Communications • Le Bonheur Children's Hospital
50 N. Dunlap, Memphis, Tennessee 38103 • (901) 287-6030 • www.lebonheur.org

ISBN 978-0-9856541-6-0

DEDICATED TO

This book is dedicated to the men and women
who have devoted their lives to caring for
children — for the past 60 years, and
for many years to come.

FOREWORD

At a children's hospital, we often have reason to celebrate. We celebrate the miracle of new life. We celebrate the gift of healing. We celebrate the joy of returning children home to their families. And on June 15, 2012, we celebrate 60 years of providing exceptional care to the children in and around our community.

When Le Bonheur Children's opened its doors 60 years ago, we promised that those doors would always be open to any child in need. Sixty years later, we continue to make good on that promise, thanks to the unwavering dedication and selfless service of our employees, physicians, family partners, donors, volunteers and supporters. The humble commitment of these individuals inspired the creation of *Once Upon a Heart* — a book of stories that chronicles 60 moments in time throughout our hospital's history.

At Le Bonheur, we work side by side with heroes every day, and we stand on the shoulders of giants. *Once Upon a Heart* is both a celebration of our hospital's first 60 years and a tribute to the people of Le Bonheur. As we continue to grow and evolve, furthering the field of pediatric medicine and deepening our commitment to our patients and families, we hope to preserve the legacy of those who have come before us. Their stories — funny, gratifying, energizing, humbling and motivating — remind us of the important mission placed before us every day. We're here to take care of kids.

It is my hope that *Once Upon a Heart* will serve as an inspiration for future generations of caregivers at Le Bonheur. We are grateful for the many people who made our first 60 years possible, and we look forward to many years to come.

Meri Armour

Meri Armour
President and CEO, Le Bonheur Children's Hospital

CONTENTS

A Happy Time

My mother, Elizabeth Jordan Gilliland, is credited with giving Le Bonheur its name. Born in 1898, she was one of only a few gals in Memphis who shared the experience of having gone to college. She went to the National Cathedral School in Washington, D.C., and then attended Finch College in New York during World War I. She studied French, as proper young ladies were told to do, and she continued her French studies in Europe after the war. When she returned home to Memphis, my mother and about a half dozen other young women — all of whom had gone to college and were not yet married — set out to do something good for their community. The group's first thought was to help children in need, regardless of their race or gender. That was an important initiative to them, as they were living in a pretty bigoted time.

The main scourge for kids in those days was polio. My mother's younger brother had it as a child and walked with a limp all his life. Crippled Children's Hospital of Memphis was the facility that provided most of the care for these kids, and my mother and her friends started helping out at the hospital, visiting families and performing odd jobs. In January 1923, the women decided that their group needed a name. Recalling her French lessons, my mother suggested "Le Bonheur." Literally it

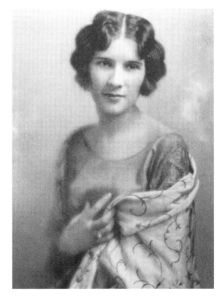

means the "good hour," but in a broad sense means "a happy time." So with unanimous agreement, the Le Bonheur Club was born.

It was a good 30 years later that the children's hospital was built. Le Bonheur Club went dormant during World War II, but after the war, it had a fresh new beginning, and in 1952, the hospital came.

Even in her later years, my mother always attended the club's annual luncheons. She would be introduced by the hospital's president, and he would always recognize her and express appreciation for what her club had done to give rise to the hospital. With a sparkle in her eye, she'd reply, "Oh, no. Thank you, but we deserve no credit. That belongs to all of you for the wonderful hospital here at Le Bonheur." She always used the French pronunciation of the name. She never said it how we do today.

My mother lived to be 97 years old. When she died, she left some money to Le Bonheur to preserve its history and support the organization. My mother loved Le Bonheur and always felt very strongly about its mission — that the hospital doors will never be closed to any child in need.

Jim Gilliland, Sr., and his wife, Lucia, are longtime friends of Le Bonheur and supporters of the Memphis community. One of the founders of Glankler Brown, Jim is an attorney who has chaired the Board of Trustees of LeMoyne Owen College, the Memphis Arts Council, the M.K. Gandhi Institute, the Cotton Carnival and the Liberty Bowl, which he helped bring to Memphis. Lucia has served as president of the Junior League, chair of the Orpheum restoration project and chair of the Center City Commission.

Four-Legged Therapist

I've been bringing my golden retriever, Kicker, to Le Bonheur for eight years. Kicker is a pet therapy dog. He spends time with patients in the lobby and up on the floors, helps to distract kids when they are getting IVs, visits families at FedExFamilyHouse and makes everyone smile.

One afternoon, Kicker and I were visiting patients up on the 10th floor with Dana from Child Life. We came around to a room with a little girl who must have been about 3 or 4 years old. She was a precious little girl who had suffered some severe burns, and she had bandages on her legs. The bottoms of her feet weren't burned, but she was afraid to put them down and walk because her burns were so painful. In order for her to go home, she had to walk around, but she just wanted to be carried.

The nurses were excited that Kicker was there and that we were going to visit this patient. They thought it would be very good medicine for her. We went in the room to see this little girl. She didn't really want to pet Kicker; she just wanted to look at him. I asked if she wanted to go for a walk, and

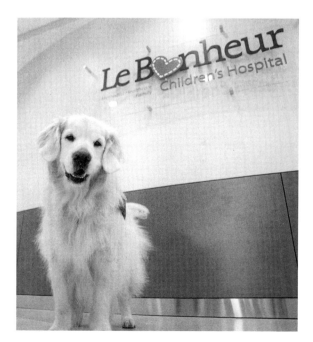

she said no. So, we mostly talked with her parents and grandparents (there were lots of family members visiting), and they told us the patient had been depressed and upset for most of her stay. You could tell by looking that this little girl had a beautiful smile, but she wouldn't smile.

When we started to leave the room, the little girl started crying and reaching for Kicker. I asked again if she wanted to go for a walk, and this time she said yes. I put a short, red leash on Kicker that's just the right size for kids, and her parents set her down. She picked up the leash and took a tentative step toward Kicker. She walked out of the room and took a few steps down the hallway, and a smile spread across her face. After a short distance, we tried to turn back, but the girl said no; she wanted to keep walking. She ended up walking Kicker all the way around the unit.

Everyone was crying, and I had goose bumps. This was the first time this patient had done anything the whole time she was in the hospital. When she was leading Kicker, she overcame her fear of walking again after her injury.

This experience reinforced how special the pet therapy program is and how Le Bonheur has been progressive by allowing patients who can't leave their rooms to have pet therapy visits on the inpatient floors. I'm not a doctor or a nurse, but thanks to Kicker, we were able to help heal this child.

People ask me how long I've been volunteering at Le Bonheur, and I tell them Kicker is the volunteer, not me. I'm just along for the ride.

Jo Anne Fusco and Kicker have been a pet therapy team for eight years. Jo Anne's other dog, Boss, has been visiting Le Bonheur for almost two years. Boss loves performing tricks for patients, including teaching kids how to stop, drop and roll.

Outside the Resus Room

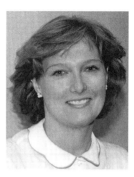

In the spring of 1983, I was 24 years old and working as a brand new nurse in the Emergency Department. I'd been in the ED for a couple of months, and I was assigned as the nurse for the trauma room. Back then, we had one trauma room, which we referred to as the resus room. The toughest cases went through this room, and I hated it because we never knew what to expect.

One afternoon, we received word that a newborn baby was on the way to the ED by ambulance. The child had been in a "car bite," which was our term for a motor vehicle accident. The paramedics brought in this precious baby boy, probably 6 weeks old, who had gone through the windshield and suffered severe head trauma. We worked on this baby for two or three hours, and he would come back — we would get a heartbeat — and then he would code again.

My role was to go out periodically and talk to the father, telling him how his son was doing. The child's mother was at the Med being treated for injuries from the wreck. When I spoke with him, the father told me that he and his wife were an older couple. They had not expected to have this baby, but the child had infused their home with energy and new life.

After a few hours spent trying to revive the baby, the doctor determined that there was nothing more we could do, and the child was pronounced dead. It was my job to go out and give the news to the father.

I was sobbing so hard I couldn't speak. I brought the baby out so the father could hold his child and have some closure with his son. I sat down with him, and we just cried together for awhile.

At the time, I felt like a failure. As a new nurse, I really questioned whether I was doing anyone any good because I was so upset about the death of this child. I felt horrible for this family that they had lost their baby, and I was upset that I had not controlled my emotions.

And then, the next day, a huge basket of fruit was delivered to the Emergency Department. It was addressed to me with a note from the father, and the note read, "Thank you for caring for our baby."

The father's tender gesture during this fragile time made me realize that it was OK to cry with the family. It was OK to show them my human side as well as my caretaker side, and it helped me to know that it meant something to this family when they saw how much I cared about their son. When I was 24, I saw my job as monitoring patients, administering medications and performing clinical duties. Now, as a mother, I have a better understanding of what our time together may have meant to this father.

Jennilyn Jennings Utkov worked as a nurse at Le Bonheur for two years before returning to school to pursue a master's degree in marketing. She now serves as Le Bonheur's administrative director of Marketing and Communications.

Original Pioneers

I came to Memphis in October of 1977 to take over the reins as president and CEO of Le Bonheur Children's — a role I ended up holding until 1995. Before moving to Memphis, my family and I lived in Washington, D.C. I recall that one of the reasons we were so excited about coming to Memphis was because we could get good barbecue and turnip greens, which we could not get in D.C.

After arriving in Memphis, I became close friends with Drs. James Etteldorf and James Hughes, known among friends as Dr. E and The General respectively. Dr. Hughes was also my backdoor neighbor. These men were the original pioneers of Le Bonheur, and they set high standards for all of us who followed. I am thankful to them for the foundation they gave to me and for the example they set for all who came after them. They never quit, and they both lived lives worth emulating.

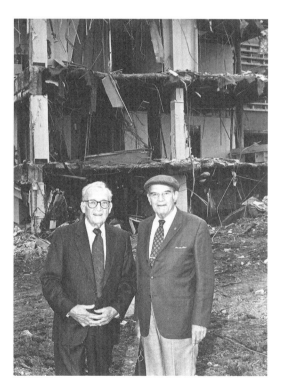

These men serve as such an inspiration to me that, to this day, I keep photographs of them in my office to remind myself of their sacrifices. The pictures show them standing in front of the original 1952 Le Bonheur when it was torn down in 1980 to add on to the building.

Drs. Etteldorf and Hughes held the banner high and established the standards of excellence Le Bonheur still adheres to today. For me, what Le Bonheur comes down to is that all of us share the same passion and commitment to restoring children who are sick or injured to the highest possible level of health. This is accomplished in part because everyone who works for Le Bonheur loves kids. 🤍

Gene Cashman is CEO of The Urban Child Institute. He served at the helm of Le Bonheur Children's Medical Center from 1977 to 1995.

A Grand Event

We first announced to our Associates that we were planning to build a new hospital in 2005. Thanks to gifts from The Urban Child Institute and other donors, we had already raised more than $56 million for the new Le Bonheur. As we announced the plan to build, a group of children turned over big blocks that showed how much money had already been raised. My son, Ronald, 12, was one of the kids holding a block. I remember he seemed a little nervous, but afterward he was excited about meeting the other kids and taking part in the big day. We still have a sticker on our fridge at home that says "Ronald — Le Bonheur Ambassador."

After demolition began on the Memphis Mental Health Institute — the site for the new Le Bonheur — we would eat lunch in the Human Resources break room every day and watch the building come down. Our offices are at the corner of Poplar Avenue and Dunlap Street, so we had a front row seat to the demolition. We

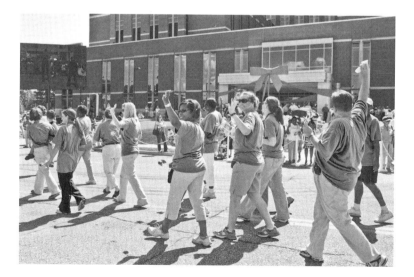

always heard lots of clanging and banging, and on two different occasions, we heard a big "POOF!" sound and then saw a giant cloud of dust coming toward us across Poplar. We'd see the cloud and start to worry, but then we'd realize something big had just come down, and the dust was settling.

Eventually, we had a clear view from our office across to the old Le Bonheur, and then we watched the new building go up. Watching the construction was a favorite pastime of ours for several years. We formed a new respect, too, for the people outside working in the heat and the cold.

On June 15, 2010, we held a grand opening celebration for the new Le Bonheur. I was on the planning committee. Even though planning for an event like that can be overwhelming at times, the group was great about sharing ideas and listening to everyone's opinions. Being part of this particular day — out there in the crowd seeing the smiles on the staff, doctors' and kids' faces — was pretty amazing.

We held a parade before the actual ceremony, and before the parade started, Shirley Catron and I sat in the back parking lot of the Physicians' Office Building passing out sunscreen and pop-up books. Other people were passing out fans and bottles of water. My son, Randall, volunteered to march in the parade group with the little kids. I'd bought him a little spray bottle fan, and he walked around spraying the kids to help keep them cool. He felt like a hero. Shirley and I walked in the parade with the staff float. We tried to make it fun by doing a dance, getting the crowd involved and getting them up on their feet. Standing up, clapping, yelling and cheering — anything we could do to get our minds off the hot day, we did it.

At the end of the ceremony, Meri Armour and Gary Shorb stood with a group of children, and they untied a giant ribbon on the front of the hospital. Each of the kids looked so determined to do a good job pulling the ribbon. They had so much energy, and it was just great. It truly was a grand event and a great memory for Le Bonheur. 🤍

Rachel Booker has worked at Le Bonheur Children's for 21 years as a Human Resources generalist. She currently resides in Memphis with her family.

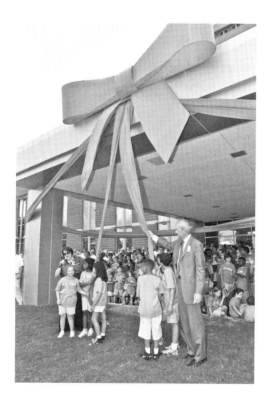

Three of a Kind

My sisters and I were the first set of identical triplets ever born in Tipton County. We were brought into this world on June 5, 1956 — almost two months before we were expected.

As our father, Harold, tells it, our mother, Margaret Ann, went into labor on a weekend. We lived in the small rural farm community of Burlison, Tenn. — not quite 10 miles from Covington — and the local doctor's office was closed. There was no hospital

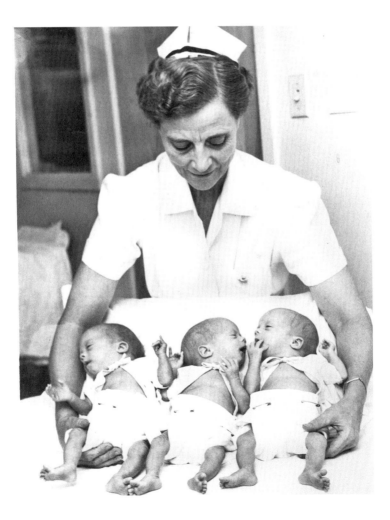

nearby. So a Covington physician, Dr. Norman L. Hyatt, opened his office and turned an examination room into a makeshift delivery room. Our aunt, Nellene, traveled to Covington with our parents and assisted Dr. Hyatt, administering ether to our mother during the birth.

No one knew she would be having triplets.

As Dr. Hyatt delivered first me, then my sister Marty and finally our sister Elaine, he laid us under an old-fashioned crookneck lamp for warmth. Each of us weighed only about 3 pounds, and Elaine — the smallest of the three — weighed only 2 pounds, 13 ounces.

After wrapping us in blankets, Dr. Hyatt called the local funeral home because there was no ambulance in the area. A hearse arrived with the heater turned up as high as it would go — even though it was June and already very hot outside. Our father, Aunt Nell and the three of us were rushed to Le Bonheur Children's Hospital, 40 miles away. Our mother was taken to a family member's home nearby to recover.

Marty, Elaine and I spent the first three months of our lives at Le Bonheur. Our parents traveled to and from Memphis every few days to see us, though they couldn't hold or even touch us. When we each reached a weight of 5 pounds, we finally went home.

Our parents went through about 36 cloth diapers a day, and they assigned us each a different colored diaper pin — green for me, blue for Marty and yellow for Elaine — so they could tell us apart. Little did they know that as we grew older, we would often dress alike, swap classes and play other pranks to keep people from guessing who was who.

My sisters and I have been inseparable since the day we were born. Every year on June 6, we celebrate our birthday together. When we turned 50, we spent the day in Memphis, touring Graceland, visiting the Memphis Zoo and dining at the Hard Rock Café on Beale Street. We also visited Le Bonheur, paying tribute to the place that saved our lives. If it hadn't been for Le Bonheur, we wouldn't be here today.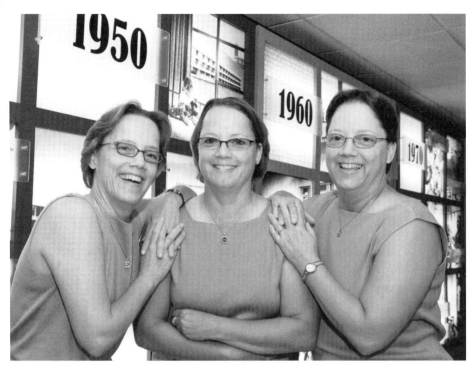

From left to right, Elaine McCommon O'Brien, Marty McCommon Turner and Jean McCommon Peeler have been celebrating their birthday together since 1956.

Comfort Zone

In the summer of 2008, I was away on business and received a call one night that my two sons were fighting for their lives at Le Bonheur. They had suffered wounds to their throats, wrists and stomachs. My younger son, Hudson, was only 11 months old at the time. His brother, Nolan, was 3.

The next morning, I walked into Le Bonheur's Pediatric Intensive Care Unit for the first time and saw how critically injured my oldest son was. A PICU nurse was rubbing Nolan's head with a wet sponge, and she looked at me and said, "He's resting really well. I just gave him a bath, and he smiled." It still brings tears to my eyes today to think about that moment. It was very surreal, just like an angel was there with him.

Nolan spent three months at Le Bonheur, and my family and I were able to stay by his bedside around the clock. The staff would hug my mother, my aunt and uncle and tell us, "We're doing everything we can, and everything is going to be OK."

One day, a nurse who had never even met us brought Nolan a Nerf basketball goal set. He attached it to the end of Nolan's bed, so he could shoot while he was recovering. This was someone who didn't know us. He just understood the trauma of the situation and, on his own time and with his own money, bought something for Nolan out of the kindness of his heart. It was clear to me that we were experiencing a different world of health care.

In early September, Nolan was fully healed and able to leave the hospital. Hudson had stayed in Intensive Care for the first two months in a medically induced coma so his wounds could heal. After that, he was transferred to the Transitional Care Unit. Le Bonheur helped us get a room at the Westin hotel downtown, where Nolan stayed with family members during the day while I was at work. After work, I would spend time with Hudson and then go to the Westin, so I could be with Nolan. Having my boys close together was the biggest help I could ever imagine.

When Hudson was ready to come home, I was scared. The hospital had become a comfort zone for me during the boys' healing. Because I am not a nurse or a doctor, I was very scared that I wouldn't be able to take care of them and that something bad would happen on my watch. Le Bonheur connected us with a social services group that helped me with Hudson's medication, oxygen levels, tracheotomy and everything that needed to be done for several weeks until I got comfortable with the process. The boy's nurses would also come by the house to check on them out of the goodness of their hearts. Having the nurses come by was very comforting and gave me a bit of confidence in what I was doing. It meant a lot.

Le Bonheur provided as much psychological care as they did medical services for my boys. Our situation was particularly traumatic because the children's wounds had been inflicted by their mother. It was almost beyond traumatic. But every nurse, the

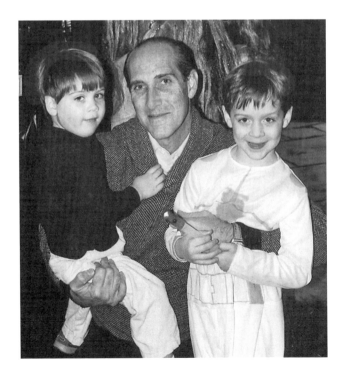

Environmental Services workers and anyone we came in contact with would tell us they were praying for us. It made me realize the hospital was there to help us in every way it could. The people at Le Bonheur didn't just save my children's lives — they also saved mine.

Rob Joyner lives in Memphis with his two sons. The boys still have a relationship with their Le Bonheur team and are healthy, active children.

The Boss Is Not at Home

In 1963, I graduated from The University of Tennessee College of Pharmacy and came to work at Le Bonheur.

The Pharmacy in those days looked like any other local drugstore. As such, we sold all the sundry items, but our biggest mover was children's toys. The actual pharmacy was located in a small section at the back of the drugstore. We were a three-pharmacist operation.

One day — I believe this was in 1964 — an agent from the Bureau of Alcohol, Tobacco and Firearms came by to make the annual inspection of alcohol. Alcohol in those days was more controlled than narcotics due to tax revenues, and these inspections were always unannounced. The measurement was made by inserting a yardstick into a 54-gallon drum of ethyl alcohol. The director — called the chief pharmacist back then — was the only one with the keys.

I asked the agent to go to our snack bar and have a cup of coffee while we waited for the director to come in. I then ran to a phone and called the boss at home to tell him the alcohol inspector was here. There was no answer. I was close to panic; this was a big deal.

The agent eventually tired of waiting and went to see the hospital administrator, who called me to see what was going on. I told him the boss was not answering his phone. He told me to send Jerry, our delivery man, to the boss's house to get him. Jerry, who didn't know about the ATF agent, came back from the errand and told me, "The boss says he is not at home."

By then, I was really in a panic. But finally, the director walked in the front door. I was so glad to see him, thinking my problems would soon be over. I will never forget this sight. The boss walked in, taking off his jacket, but as soon as I started briefing him on the alcohol agent, he stopped and started putting his jacket back on. He began backing out the door and simply said, "You haven't seen me."

It was like rewinding a scene from a movie — watching him walk forward, then backward, taking off his jacket and then putting it back on.

I never saw the director again. The next day, the hospital administrator asked me if I wanted to be the chief pharmacist. And that's how I became the boss.

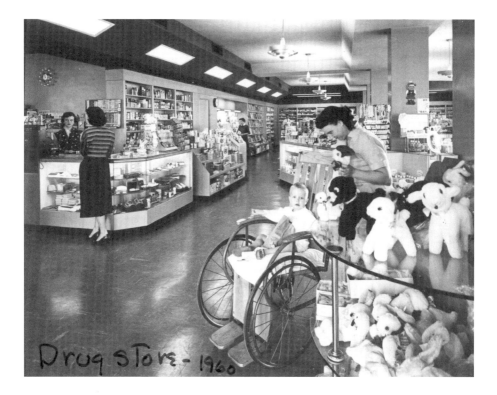

Bert Price worked in the Le Bonheur Pharmacy for 42 years until retiring as Pharmacy director in 2005.

Twins Karma

Back in the 1970s, my grandmother — Elizabeth Jordan Gilliland, who gave the Le Bonheur Club its name — would often tell me stories about the early years of the hospital. She had a very maternal attitude about Le Bonheur; she absolutely loved the place. She was also fearless. I remember once when I was about 12 years old, she took me on a trip to walk the halls and see the hospital. She was driving a 1970s Lincoln Town Car, which was about 30 feet long. My grandmother pulled into the parking lot, drove right up to the chain link fence, knocked it halfway over and hopped out of the car without batting an eyelash. She was about 80 years old at the time.

Even though I grew up with Le Bonheur, it never crossed my mind that I would ever need it for my own children. By pure chance, I was working in health care finance for Morgan Keegan in 2008 when plans to build the new Le Bonheur hospital were underway, and I was lucky to be assigned to the project. I thought that would be my Le Bonheur experience.

But in the spring of 2008 my wife, Kathryn, became pregnant with twins. For the first six months everything went well, but suddenly the pregnancy destabilized, and the twins had to be delivered terribly prematurely. The doctors told us there was only a 50/50 chance that the babies — a son, Walt, and a daughter, Jordan, named for her great-grandmother — would make it.

The twins were delivered at Methodist Germantown and spent a month in the Neonatal Intensive Care Unit there. One night, we got a call at 2 a.m. informing us that Walt had taken a dramatic turn for the worse and might not survive another 48 hours. At the same time, Jordan's lungs still had not begun working on their own, and her medical options were running out. It was a devastating time.

The next day, Walt was rushed to the Le Bonheur NICU for "hail mary" surgery. Jordan was brought to Le Bonheur shortly thereafter to be in the same room with Walt, so they could feed off of each other's "twins karma." We were on pins and needles with them both and spent countless hours at the hospital getting to know dozens of doctors, nurses and therapists.

A few weeks later, Walt turned a critical corner, and Jordan's lungs finally began to work on their own. We were beyond elated. After four grueling months in the NICU, they both made it home. Not only was medical care for the babies world class, but the staff's compassionate bedside manner made it possible to bring Walt and Jordan home with a sense of deep gratitude despite all we had been through.

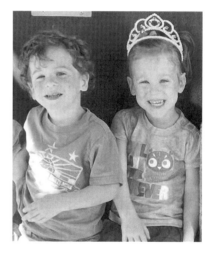

Today, Walt and Jordan are vibrant, healthy 3-year-olds. Our family couldn't be happier, and we are beyond proud that the NICU teams at Le Bonheur and Methodist Germantown call the twins the "miracle babies." I know my grandmother would be thrilled to know that the vision she and her friends helped create 60 years ago played such an important role in the lives of her loved ones. 🩶

Jim Gilliland and his wife, Kathryn, both serve on Methodist Le Bonheur's system-wide Quality Assurance Committee, as members of the Family Partners Council. They live in Memphis with their three children, Evan, age 5, and Walt and Jordan, age 3. Evan currently aspires to be a train engineer, Walt wants to be a bulldozer driver and Jordan is determined to be a ballerina when she grows up.

A Dollar A Day

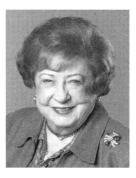

When I was 18 years old, I got my first job as a waitress in a steakhouse in Little Rock, Ark., for a dollar a day. This was in 1934 during the Depression. A few days later, my father said to me, "Mary, how much money do you make?" I said, "I make a dollar a day, and my meals and my uniforms." And he said, "Well, you know what you do with 10 cents of that dollar, don't you? You give it away." And I said, "But I only have a dollar." And he said, "Well, what if you woke up in the morning, and you had 90 cents or a dollar? What difference would it make?"

My father taught me that lesson 77 years ago — that charity is a gift for the good life we all have — and I have carried it with me throughout my life.

My husband, Herbert, who served on the Le Bonheur board of directors in the early 80s, always believed in doing for children. He believed that tackling neurological problems in the early stages could give a child an excellent chance at living a normal life.

After Herbert's death in 1985, I established a fund at Le Bonheur in support of the hospital's Neuroscience Institute. We all know that children are our future, and it's up to us to see that they have a future. And Le Bonheur has seen to that.

Mary Shainberg and her late husband, Herbert, have been among the city's leading patrons for more than two decades to champion the causes of children with developmental disorders. The Shainbergs' gifts to Le Bonheur Children's — including the Shainberg Neuroscience Research Fund — have made a significant impact for future generations.

Casting a Rope

Our son, Davis, was born Dec. 20, 2001, with a nasal defect. He was transferred to Le Bonheur Children's at 1 week old to have a trach inserted. Davis spent a little time in the Pediatric Intensive Care Unit before a three-month stay in the hospital's Special Care Unit. During that time, he developed feeding problems and an inflamed colon. When my wife and I finally brought Davis home, he had a trach, a feeding tube and required IV nutrition.

Because of our son's chronic illness, we got to know Le Bonheur and its physicians and nurses very well. Many of the staff members became our good friends, and I believe Davis became a good friend and favorite to many of the staff, as well. The people at Le Bonheur thought of the little things, as well as the big things, to make our family as comfortable as possible under the circumstances. They were advocates, good listeners, highly skilled, knowledgeable, compassionate and kind.

When Davis was 6 years old, he succumbed to his illness, and on Jan. 24, 2008, our son passed away in the PICU at Le Bonheur. We were treated with tremendous respect, warmth and support that day. And as word spread that Davis had died, many who knew him and knew our family came to the unit to give us hugs, share our tears and offer words of comfort.

Through our experience with Davis, Dana and I learned that it takes a strong partnership between the parents and the medical community to navigate the challenges of caring for a child with multiple medical needs. We wanted to give back to the Le Bonheur family in some way, so Dana and I both became members of the hospital's Family Partners Council. Dana is also now employed as an

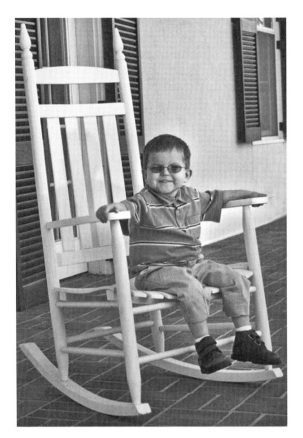

RN case manager at Le Bonheur.

In 2011, Le Bonheur nominated me for the Tennessee Hospital Association Meritorious Service Award — Individual Volunteer, and I was selected as the recipient. It was an honor to stand on stage and talk about Le Bonheur's meaningful efforts to engage parents. We are making a difference because Le Bonheur gives us a way to contribute. I feel like my opinion matters every time I walk into a meeting.

I realized something else as I waited to receive my award. I was listening to the key note speaker, Coast Guard Captain Larry Brudnicki, recall his rescue missions during the worst weather in 100 years — the perfect storm. During one mission, Brudnicki's crew rescued everyone except one airman from a crashed helicopter. The crew tried everything they could to find this airman, but eventually they realized they must return to shore or risk losing everyone else.

At that point, I realized what Le Bonheur did for Dana and me. We all worked tirelessly to save Davis, but in the end we couldn't despite our very best efforts. We were lost at sea, but in the midst of our greatest storm, the Le Bonheur family reached out and pulled us into their boat. We started rowing together. Le Bonheur gave us another way to focus our energy. It gave us a way to help others and valued our efforts to make a difference. Davis inspires us to do a little more each day to help other children and their families during their storms. Thank you, Le Bonheur, for casting a rope to us. Thank you for touching our hearts with your exceptional care.

Don Hutson and his wife, Dana, both serve on Le Bonheur's Family Partners Council. Don serves as the co-chairman of the council's Quality and Safety Committee, as well as assists with efforts to improve communication between families and the medical staff. Dana is a member of the council's Staff Education Committee, and she also works as a nurse on the hospital's Case Management team. The Hutsons reside in Memphis with their daughter, Deanna.

Strain

In 1986, I took care of a patient who was at death's door when he came to Le Bonheur. He was 3 years old, and his electrolytes were extremely imbalanced. He was very sick. After running a battery of tests, the patient was diagnosed with HIV. At that point, he had full-blown AIDS.

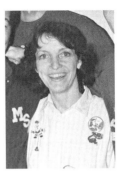

This was a different era at Le Bonheur. We didn't even have coffee pots on the units back then. There was a pharmacist who worked here in the 80s, and everyone called him Strain. He was our only night pharmacist, and folks would call down to the pharmacy in the evening and put in their coffee requests to Strain. He would brew a fresh pot and send cups of coffee up through the dumb waiter to anyone who requested it. Strain kept many of us awake and going on the night shifts.

My night shifts caring for this patient came around the same time we started teaching about precautions from blood and bodily fluids and wearing gloves consistently. At that time in nursing school, we were taught that we shouldn't wear gloves unless we knew our patient had a communicable disease in order to keep from offending anyone. We also saw a trend among hemophilia patients throughout the country. Donor centers did not test blood for HIV then, and many hemophiliacs contracted HIV through their Factor VIII and subsequently died of AIDS. It was a time of tremendous change in health care.

I took care of this little boy for a few weeks, and eventually he stabilized and reached a point where he was up and running around. This patient was one of the first participants in the St. Jude HIV treatment program.

About 15 years after I treated him, I happened to run into the social worker who currently worked with that program at St. Jude. I asked her about this boy. She knew exactly who I was talking about and told me they had been very successful in his treatment plan. He was a great young man — 18 years old, in remission, outgoing and very upbeat.

That was a wonderful moment for me — to know after all this time that he had made it. He was OK.

Ila McDonald has worked in nursing at Le Bonheur since 1984. She currently serves as GI coordinator.

Can I Come Home?

Back in the 70s, before we had good ultrasound technology, doctors and parents knew very little about a baby's condition until he or she was born. If a child was born with a defect, but there wasn't something immediately and obviously wrong, often the problem was not discovered until later in infancy. I was born in September 1977. I looked like a normal, healthy baby, but when I was 6 months old — up on my knees and crawling around — I started having a lot of gastrointestinal problems. I couldn't keep anything down, and my mom and dad took me to the pediatrician.

My parents were told that I had a stomach bug and just needed a day or so to recover. However, my GI issues continued. Finally, my parents brought me to the Emergency Department at Le Bonheur. Doctors there learned I had a hernia in my diaphragm, and my stomach was pushed up into that hole. I had surgery to correct the problem the next day, spent one night in the Intensive Care Unit, stayed for another night on an inpatient floor, and four days after coming to the ED, we went home. I've been better ever since. My parents always talk about how impressed they were that once they came to Le Bonheur, the problem was diagnosed and corrected so quickly.

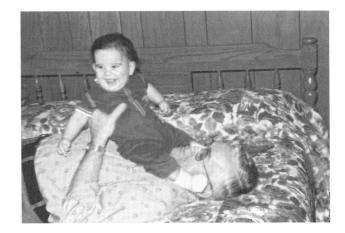

I ended up working at Le Bonheur by accident. I majored in biology in college and wanted to work in health care, so I became an EMT and a paramedic. I came to work at Le Bonheur as a stepping stone to working with the Memphis Fire Department. After three years here, I took a job as a paramedic with MFD. But after a few weeks away from Le Bonheur, I realized how much I missed working in the ED. I called my boss and said, "Please, can I come home?" Luckily, she said yes. I've been back at Le Bonheur for two years, and in all likelihood, this will be my career. I feel like this is where I'm supposed to be.

Blake Bobbitt has worked in the Le Bonheur ED for five years as an EDT III. His wife, Julie, works as a logistics specialist on the 10th floor. They live in Memphis with their 3-year-old son, Jesse.

Mugga Mugga

It was Jan. 7, 2010. School had been canceled due to snow, and my 10-year-old son, Reese, was playing at a friend's house in our neighborhood. Our youngest daughter was at the same house playing with another friend.

The phone rang. I answered, and I heard my daughter say, "Reese drowned. He's dead." All I could think was, "What is she talking about?" I asked to speak to Quinn — Reese's friend — and he told me Reese and some other boys had been playing on a frozen pond in our neighborhood. Three of them fell through the ice. Two of them had gotten out, but Reese was in the middle and couldn't get out. I heard Quinn say, "He's been under for 10 minutes."

I tore through the house and into the backyard. I didn't even know about the pond. My oldest daughter was with me, and we were running through the woods, trying to find our way to the pond. I told my daughter to go get Quinn, so he could show us, the way. Right then, I heard an ambulance. It pulled up beside us and the paramedics asked where to go. At the same moment, Quinn's grandfather came over the hill and led us all to the pond.

I saw a hole in the middle of the ice, and Reese's hat was floating in the water. He was still under, and no one knew how to get to him. I yelled, "Somebody, please go get him!"

A team of rescue workers took a boat onto the pond, and they were fishing for him, trying to find him in the water. Time stood still for me. Finally, I heard a detective say, "I got him," and they pulled him out. They wouldn't let me see him but rushed him to the ambulance. He had been under the water for more than 20 minutes.

Someone came up to me and told me Reese was on his way to Le Bonheur. They said he didn't have a heartbeat and wasn't breathing, but that the cold water was good for him. By the time I got to Le Bonheur, his heart was beating again. But Reese's lungs were severely damaged, and he still wasn't breathing. Even on a ventilator, he was only getting 20 percent oxygen. I started crying. It hit me — I could really lose him. Reese could die.

Eventually the team decided to put Reese on ECMO — a machine that provides support to the heart and lungs. A chaplain came to speak with me and asked if I needed anything. She later told me that in that moment, she was sent to prepare me for losing Reese, but something told her to wait.

We were told that Reese could be on ECMO for at least six weeks. I was preparing myself to teach him to walk again, to talk again. I was prepared for that to be my life, and I didn't care as long as I had my son. About 24 hours later, the team noticed that Reese was breathing some on his own. Even though it still wasn't enough, we knew it was a good sign. His brain was telling him to breathe.

The nurses were wonderful and patient, and they always talked to Reese like he was still there, saying things like, "I'm going to reach over you now." By the third day, Reese started responding. He squeezed my husband's hand, wiggled his feet on command, and at that point, I knew I'd have him back. It was just a matter of time.

Less than a week later, he was off the ventilator and breathing on his own. One night when my husband came to the hospital and I was heading home, I leaned in to kiss Reese on the forehead, and he mumbled something that I couldn't quite hear. I said, "What, buddy," and leaned in. "Mugga mugga," he repeated. He was referencing our nightly ritual — mugga mugga, hug hug, kiss kiss — when we would rub noses, hug and kiss before bed.

Two weeks after he fell through the ice, Reese walked out of Le Bonheur. It took him a while to regain his physical health and strengthen his cognitive skills, but most things you wouldn't even notice unless you knew his personality. For the first few months after he came home, Reese cried at night, saying "I'm so thankful. I'm here. I'm alive." He knows how close he came to death.

We go visit the staff at Le Bonheur each year around the holidays. I have followed stories about other children who have fallen through the ice and not survived, or who have survived but with brain damage or a lack of mobility. And then I look at my son who is healthy and whole, and I think, "Why us? Why Reese?" I am humbled and blessed. ♥

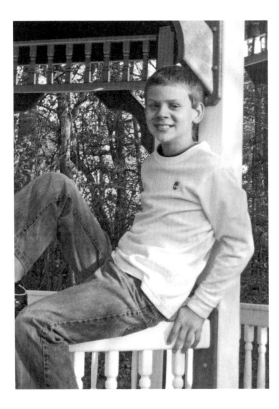

Tracey Wagner lives in Bartlett, Tenn., with her husband, Aaron, and their three children. Reese served as a grand marshal for Le Bonheur's grand opening parade in June 2010.

Thor

I n the early 90s, I worked as a night weekend nurse on 4 Central. One evening, two of our nurses found a large cricket on the sidewalk outside the hospital. They captured him, put him in a specimen cup and brought him upstairs to live on our unit. We named him Thor and quickly adopted him as our night weekender mascot.

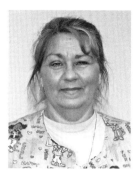

Not long after Thor came to live with us, one of the nurses got the idea to send him through the tube system in his specimen cup house to visit another unit. We included a note and sent him to a neighboring department. Soon, he came back through the system accompanied by a reply note. We sent Thor through the tube system to visit other units, and it became a ritual every weekend for him to visit each unit. At the end of the weekend, Thor would be sent home to 4 Central, and he would stay in a locker during the week.

When Thor passed away, a formal visitation was held for him on 4 Central. Our team put out a guest book, and staff from other units came by to bid farewell. A Viking boat was constructed from paper towels. The nurses put Thor in the paper towel boat, sprinkled him with glitter and gave him a Viking funeral at sea.

In the midst of our late-night shifts, sharing visits from Thor with other units was a stress reliever and boosted camaraderie among our teams.

Laura Luther has worked at Le Bonheur Children's since 1986. She currently serves as a patient care coordinator on the 12th floor.

Never Hurt Me

In the early 1980s, I was working as a nurse in the Pediatric Intensive Care Unit. A 13-year-old girl was admitted to the PICU with a severe and rapidly progressive disease process. She remained in our unit for 10 months. Despite her treatment, this patient routinely bled out, and we took her to surgery repeatedly. It was very difficult to take care of her. She was in a lot of pain, and she constantly wanted someone at her bedside. Her situation was so difficult that many nurses didn't want to be assigned to her, so I took care of her almost every day that I worked over the course of that year. Over time, she and I became very good friends.

During her hospitalization, someone gave this patient a white kitten. She'd never seen it — only pictures that her parents brought. In fact, she had never seen a white kitten at all. She became very fixated on that cat and often talked about wanting to see him and hold him.

So one day, I stopped by her parents' house, picked up the cat, put it in a cardboard box and smuggled it into the hospital. I did my best to stick to isolated hallways and back stairwells, and I made it to the unit. Then lo and behold, who happened to be on the unit at that moment but the chief nursing officer! She was making rounds, walking from room to room. I kept pace behind her, so that when she was on one side of the unit, I was on the other. The PICU was an open unit at that time, but this patient was in one of the private rooms. Soon I was able to sneak into her room with the kitten. She only spent about four or five minutes with the cat, but after that, it was all she ever talked about.

Eventually, she started to get well. After she was discharged, she would come back periodically for various tests and procedures. Any time she returned for a procedure, she would have her parents call me, and I would always be the one to insert her IV, catheter, feeding tube or whatnot. It began to bother me that I was always the one who did painful procedures to her. Finally one day I asked her, "Why do you always ask for me to do these painful things?" She looked up at me with an expression of pure surprise and said, "Because I know you love me; you would never intentionally hurt me."

What I remember most about my time at Le Bonheur is not the friends I have made, although I have many, but the patients I cared for. I remember so many of their names and their stories, which are now part of my life. Each child is a unique creation, and I am overwhelmed by the trust that parents place in us each day to treasure them and protect them. We come here to do the right thing for our kids.

Elesia Turner has worked at Le Bonheur Children's since 1979. She worked as a nurse in the PICU from 1979-1993. Since 1993, she has served as a clinical educator, PICU clinical director, nursing administrator of the Emergency Department and patient safety officer. She currently holds the role of director of Risk Management.

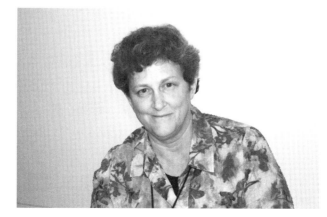

A Pretty Good Fellow

<hr>

In 1956, I was living in Milan, Tenn. I had worked at the Arsenal for about five years and felt like it was time to move on. I lived with two other girls; my roommates had both gotten jobs in Memphis. I saw an ad in the *The Commercial Appeal* for a job working at Le Bonheur as an administrative secretary, and I thought it sounded interesting, so I wrote a letter to inquire about the job. I had a response, went on an interview and was hired. The three of us moved to Memphis and got a place together out east. Our next-door neighbors introduced me to a lady named Alice "Pat" Patton who worked at Le Bonheur, and Pat quickly became my very best friend. I worked at the hospital as the secretary to Al Dierks, the administrator. I enjoyed my work, and the time passed quickly.

After I had been at Le Bonheur for about three years, one of Pat's friends — a gentleman named N.W. Tucker — decided to introduce me to a friend of his, Faser Triplett. Faser was a pediatric resident at John Gaston Hospital and rotated at Le Bonheur. N.W. and Pat lived in the same apartment building, and they set up a time for Faser and me to meet. The four of us got together and had a nice visit, and then a week or two later, Faser invited me to go to a Tennessee game in Knoxville with him and some of his friends.

I went to the football game, and on the way home, I prayed that I would never have to go out with him again. His friends were kind of put out that he took me to the game because he had been dating some other girl not long before, and they were standoffish with me. When I got home, I thought, "That was the worst time I have ever had in my life."

But after a day or two, he called me, and we went out again, and then we started going out a lot. He was more fun than anybody I had ever known. I met all of the outstanding interns and residents from John Gaston and Le Bonheur. There was a place at John Gaston called The Pavilion where all the residents lived, and we went to the most fun parties there. We had a great time together.

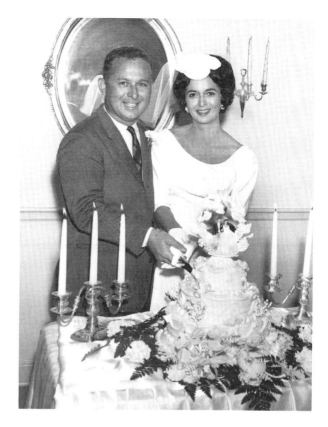

I also got to experience how wonderful Faser was with little children. The front of my office was open to the main hallway — with swinging doors — so I could see everything that happened up and down the hall. I would see him walking down the hall with these little children perched on his shoulders, and he was so tender and sweet with them that I thought, "Well, he's a pretty good fellow after all."

After he finished his residency, Faser decided to join the Air Force. I was just heartbroken that he was going to leave. The summer before he enlisted, he moved to Clarksdale, Miss., to work for the Health Department. One day that summer, the phone rang at Le Bonheur. It was Faser on the other end, and he said, "Since I'm leaving to go into the service, will you marry me?" I said yes, and we decided to get married that fall on my birthday — Sept. 28 — to help him remember our anniversary.

We married in September of 1961, and then he immediately went off to The Flight Surgeon School. Mr. Dierks didn't want me to leave Memphis right away, so I stayed and worked for another month, and then I moved to San Antonio. We lived in Texas for two years and had a little boy and a little girl in Abilene, so when we came home to Memphis, we brought back two Texans and a dog.

Faser completed his fellowship as an allergist at Le Bonheur, and after that, we moved to Jackson, Miss., where he became the first board-certified allergist in the state. That was the end of our time at Le Bonheur, but we have always been grateful to Le Bonheur for helping us find each other. ♥

Jackie and Faser Triplett were married for almost 49 years. Faser passed away in 2010, and Jackie currently resides in Jackson, Miss. They have one son, four daughters, and 10 grandchildren who all live in Jackson.

Here's My Card

L e Bonheur saved my son Shane's life twice. When he was only 4 months old, Shane developed a rare form of epilepsy that caused severe spasms and diminished his growth and development. Doctors at Le Bonheur were able to arrest these spasms through the use of experimental drug therapies, and Shane's disorder was cured within a matter of months.

Then, at age 4, Shane was airlifted to Le Bonheur after a routine tonsillectomy at an adult outpatient hospital left him with a collapsed lung. After spending several days in Le Bonheur's Pediatric Intensive Care Unit and another few days on an inpatient floor, Shane went home with a clean bill of health. With such wonderful outcomes for my special little guy, I was happy to join Le Bonheur's Family Partners Council — a group that helps the hospital focus on providing family-centered care.

In 2010, I became chair of the council's Advocacy and Public Policy Committee. The committee works to educate and engage families and public policy officials on child health issues. My family and I traveled to Washington, D.C., in July 2011 to represent Le Bonheur at the National Association of Children's Hospitals and Related Institutions Family Advocacy Days. We were among 25 families from across the country selected to meet with legislators and share our stories on Capitol Hill.

On the morning of our visit to the Hill, our first appointment was with Congressman Steve Cohen. Shane, 5 years old, was a little apprehensive while sitting outside his office. But as soon as Congressman Cohen welcomed us inside, Shane was entranced by the Memphis memorabilia and decided the congressman was a pretty cool guy. He grasped Cohen's hand firmly, shook it vigorously and quickly uttered, "Hi, I'm Shane Casey from Memphis, Tenn., and Le Bonheur Children's Hospital saved my life twice! Here's my card!"

Congressman Cohen chuckled and took the card, and he and Shane sat down on the sofa together and talked at length. Shane readily accepted Cohen's offer to sit behind his desk while I shared our story. When it was time to go, Shane shook Cohen's hand and thanked him, then straightened his suit coat and walked out a new little man.

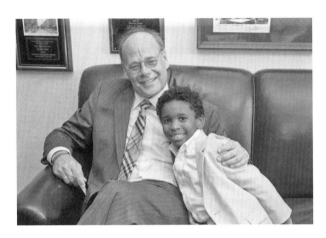

As we began to move from office to office, Shane became a real pro at introducing himself and talking about how much he loved Le Bonheur. Upon meeting Sen. Bob Corker, Shane shook his hand, said his speech and stayed at the board table with the adults to discuss Le Bonheur in more depth. After making sure we had captured his visit with the senator on film, Shane asked, "Who will I meet with next?"

Later that afternoon, we met with health care advisors from Sen. Lamar Alexander and Congressman Marsha Blackburn's offices. Just as we were ending our meeting with Blackburn's advisor, Congressman Blackburn ran from the House floor back to her office just to meet our family. Shane immediately turned to her, shook her hand earnestly and delivered his lines. To our surprise, the Congressman continued shaking Shane's hand and introduced herself in the exact same manner! We all laughed, and Shane and his little sister gave her a huge hug.

It was an honor to represent Le Bonheur as an advocate for children's health care. As a parent, it is comforting to know that Le Bonheur truly values and listens to its patients and families.

Tiffany Casey lives in Cordova, Tenn., with her two children, Shane and Bradley. She continues to serve on the Family Partners Council's Advocacy Committee.

Evolution

I came to Le Bonheur in 1987 as chair of the Department of Pediatrics for The University of Tennessee. I graduated from medical school in 1968 and eventually became a pediatric nephrologist. Medicine has changed quite a bit since I first started practicing.

I've seen great change in the medications available for children. More drugs are now tested on children, so children's doses are better evaluated. For so long, there was this idea that testing medicine on children was harmful, so it wasn't done. In reality, what we've learned is that if you don't test medications on the intended audience, you harm them more. As a result, we see fewer warnings today about the lack of testing of medicines — and medical devices — for children.

The use of the modern computer has also better enabled us to diagnose and treat children. With the electronic medical record, we can access information portably and get imaging and test results in real time. In 1987, Le Bonheur had one MRI and CT scanner, and they were relatively slow compared to today's standards. Advances in technology also give us the ability to statistically and epidemiologically analyze large patient data sets, which helps advance pediatric medicine.

Technology and procedures such as laparoscopy have improved our tests and even surgeries, and we are able to use more minimally invasive methods on children. Because of that, we are able to treat children more often in an outpatient setting. That technology has often improved our genetic testing, and we are able to test for viruses in real time now.

I've also seen an evolution in the diseases we treat. Largely because of vaccines, we no longer see children with *H. influenza* meningitis, nor as much rotovirus or pneumococcal disease. HIV isn't a death sentence anymore, and we can detect, prevent and manage the disease better for children. We have also seen great advances in treating cystic fibrosis, children's cancer, renal disease, asthma

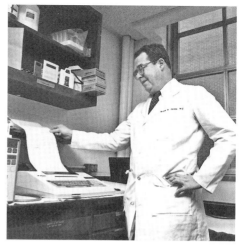

and diabetes. On the flip side, we've seen the emergence of new conditions such as obesity, type 2 diabetes and vitamin D deficiency.

There has also been a great cultural shift — both in the students I train and the families I see. We see far more female pediatricians and surgeons than before, and Le Bonheur employs more male nurses, social workers and therapists than in years past. With the patient population, we see more and more families from Africa, Eastern Europe and Latino countries. Our work force and our city are evolving.

In June 2010, we moved into a brand new facility — another sign of progress and change. I was stationed in the command center throughout the transition. Everything was so well engineered and organized. Even though there were a thousand tiny glitches, none of them mattered. The move experience showed me how incredibly well the Le Bonheur team works together. There was such symmetry to it and so much team building. The whole experience is an incredible memory for me.

Russell Chesney is a pediatric nephrologist and has worked at Le Bonheur Children's since 1987. In 2011, he won the John Howland award — the highest honor of the American Pediatric Society. Dr. Chesney lives in Memphis with his wife, Joan, who is also a physician.

At Our Fingertips

Our oldest son, John Shields Wilson, was born in the fall of 1993. He appeared to be a happy, healthy baby. But within a few hours of coming home from the hospital, John Shields was spitting up liquid with a mustardy consistency. It didn't look right, so my wife, Susan, and I took him to the pediatrician.

We were incredibly fortunate that our pediatrician, Dr. Ed Perry, realized right away that we needed to get to Le Bonheur. At

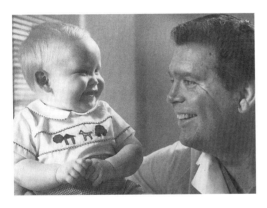

Le Bonheur, a barium X-ray revealed that John Shields had a blockage — a twisted intestine that was preventing him from digesting anything. The physician, Dr. Bob Hollabaugh, came in to tell us that the blood supply had been cut off, and John Shields needed to have surgery immediately. Bob said that if they could not get in there and untwist the intestine in time, the diagnosis was not compatible with life.

John Shields was rushed to an operating room, and my wife and I made a few phone calls to bring some heavy-duty praying to bear. One of the calls was to my wife's brother, a doctor in Decatur, Ala. He said, "If this was happening to me, there's no place I'd rather have my child than at Le Bonheur." We felt like we were in the best possible hands given the situation.

We'd been in the waiting room no more than 15 minutes or so when a nurse came out and told us the problem had been caught in time. Dr. Hollabaugh untwisted the intestine, and it pinked right up. Our son was going to be OK.

After he came out of surgery, John Shields spent about a week recovering in the Special Care Unit. I sat by his bed from 6 p.m. until 6 a.m. for a solid week; my wife and I wanted someone sitting with him around the clock.

When he was almost 2, Le Bonheur asked if they could nominate John Shields as the Children's Miracle Network Child of the Year. He was selected as Tennessee's CMN Child of the Year, so we were flown to Washington, D.C., where we went to the White House and met with Hillary Clinton. We then flew to Orlando and took part in the CMN telethon.

Susan and I realized on that trip that ours was one of only a few truly happy outcomes. John Shields is a great athlete and is preparing to go to college next year, and he has a wonderful life because we had a place like Le Bonheur available to us. I guess if you've never had to go through something as traumatic as this, you don't really realize what it means to have Le Bonheur right here at our fingertips. But for us, it means everything.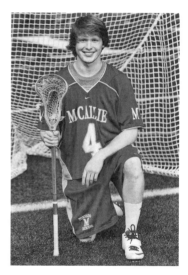

John Wilson and his wife, Susan, live in Chattanooga, Tenn., with their two sons. John Shields Wilson is 18 years old and plans to attend college in the fall.

No Substitute

Ever since I was knee high to a duck, I knew I wanted to be a pediatrician. I'm not really sure why — I didn't even have a pediatrician back then — but it was intuition. I just knew that's what I wanted to do. I graduated from medical school in 1939 and became a pediatric resident in Memphis. There were a couple of fellows who were older than me, and I did all their dirty work and made their house calls. On Sundays, we would make house calls all afternoon. I had a convertible, so we'd put the top down, and my children would ride around with me. I kept a glove and catcher's mitt in the car, and they'd pitch ball while I was inside with the patient.

Back then, we all talked about needing a children's hospital. We were excited about the idea. Before Le Bonheur, when we had a pediatric patient, we had to send them to one of the adult hospitals. My office was near Methodist, so I sent most of my patients to Methodist. My wife, Louise, was in the Le Bonheur Club during those years. Le Bonheur Club was big stuff. Those women told us what to do, and we did it.

I admitted the very first patient to Le Bonheur when it opened in 1952 — a little girl with nephritic

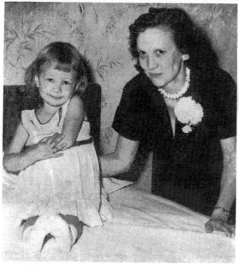

MONDAY JUNE 23, 1952 **Memphis Press-Scimitar**

PATTY AND HER MOTHER—The 3-year-old Philadelphia, Miss., miss became the first patient at the new Le Bonheur Children's Hospital today. —Press-Scimitar Staff Photo by Ralph Armstrong

Patty, Age 3, Is the Very First Patient At Le Bonheur Children's Hospital

syndrome from Tupelo, Miss. We admitted her and put her on the third floor, right by the nurses' desk. We put her on steroids for 10 days, and she got well and went on home to Tupelo. It was almost like magic when we gave steroids.

When the hospital first opened, it had about 90 beds. Most of the rooms were double rooms. We had quite a bit of polio back then. I recall once we had four iron lungs at Le Bonheur at one time, but we saw a little bit of everything. Occasionally we had diphtheria, which was sort of unheard of. But my specialty was skin and its contents; I treated everything.

I had some really sick kids at Le Bonheur over the years. You always remember your very sick ones. Some of them you didn't expect to get well, but they got well. Doctors from out of town would refer patients to me. I knew most all of the docs, and they'd send children to me. At the children's hospital, we were used to taking care of kids. There's no substitute for that.

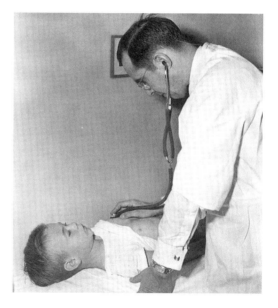

Dr. Charlie Housholder practiced pediatric medicine until retiring at age 70. He and his wife, Louise, currently reside in Germantown, Tenn.

Lean on Our Faith

In 2000, when I was 4 years old, I had a liver transplant at Le Bonheur. I hadn't been feeling well for about a week, and in church one morning, my mom realized that I just didn't look right. She took me to see my pediatrician, and when I still didn't get better, they sent me to Le Bonheur's Emergency Department.

At Le Bonheur, Dr. John Eshun determined that I needed a liver transplant. The doctors still aren't sure what caused my liver to fail — maybe a virus, they said. But I needed a new liver.

Several family members and friends volunteered to get their blood tested and see if they could donate part of their liver. My mom and dad didn't have the right blood type, but my uncle, John Monaghan, had a matching blood type and was deemed to be young enough and in good shape. He says he would have been offended if the doctors hadn't picked him.

Just four days after we arrived at Le Bonheur, I got a liver transplant. I was at Le Bonheur for three weeks recovering from surgery, and after that, I was in and out of the hospital for about a year. It seemed like every holiday, I would get sick and have to come

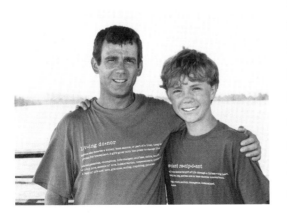

back to Le Bonheur. I never went back to the Pediatric Intensive Care Unit, but I spent several nights with IV antibiotics and had to have a liver biopsy once to make sure things were OK. Now, I have a check up every quarter with Dr. Eshun.

I still take medicine and will for the rest of my life, but it doesn't bother me.

I was so young when I got the transplant that I only remember some of it, but I am reminded of that time through pictures and stories. My mom tells me that after the surgery, the surgeon came to see my family in the waiting room. He told them that they'd done all they could, and I was in God's hands. She says that when she thinks back on that time, she should have been more scared, but for some reason, she felt really comfortable. The surgeon was telling us that they had given me their absolute best, and now we all had to lean on our faith.

My parents were there when I opened my eyes after surgery. My mom asked me if I needed anything, and I asked for a Rice Krispie treat. That's when they knew I was their same little boy, she said. They knew I was going to be OK.

When I came home from the hospital, there was a surprise party for me and an inflatable gorilla in my front yard. For a 4-year-old, that's about as good as it gets.

To me, Le Bonheur means giving second chances to kids who then have opportunities to make the world a better place. Le Bonheur saves lives.

Robert Gooch is a 16-year-old high school student. He plays lacrosse at school and recently traveled to Italy on a study abroad program. He and his uncle, John, made Le Bonheur history as the hospital's first living donor split liver transplant.

I Was Determined

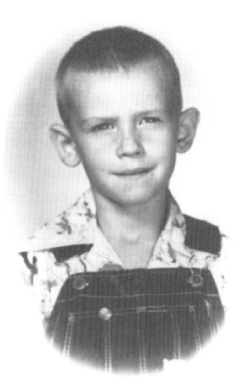

My experience at Le Bonheur happened more than 50 years ago, but I still remember going through the hospital's Emergency Department doors like it was yesterday. I was in fifth grade at the time and had been mowing my elderly neighbor's lawn in my hometown of Medina, Tenn., when I blacked out.

My parents were scared, and they rushed me straight to a clinic in the nearby town of Alamo. That is where I was born, and my mother and father knew the doctors there. The doctors thought I had a case of appendicitis and removed my appendix, but later my parents insisted on sending me to Le Bonheur Children's Hospital in Memphis for a second opinion.

At Le Bonheur, they found I had two forms of polio. No one knew how I caught it, but it was a very contagious disease. I was placed in isolation for six weeks; it felt like an eternity. My mother stayed with me the entire time, and no one else could come in or out. My friends and relatives brought me stacks and stacks of comic books to read.

After six weeks, I was well enough to go home, but I had to be on bed rest for one year. Everything that had been in my hospital room with me — clothes, toys and my comic books — had to be burned.

I remember I had to lie flat on my back with no pillow, and I watched the other kids play outside from my bedroom window. Thanks to a teacher who came to my home, I was able to continue my school lessons and start the sixth grade on time.

After that, I saw a Memphis-based Campbell Clinic orthopedist regularly. He and my other doctors thought I'd never be able to do the same things as kids my age. But I was determined to keep up with my peers even though I had been sick. I played baseball and basketball and ran track at school just like everyone else.

I'm still determined to this day.

Curtis F. Mansfield lives in Jackson, Tenn., with his wife, Joan. He is president of FirstBank in Jackson, a board member for West Tennessee Healthcare, secretary and treasurer of the Jackson Chamber of Commerce and a member of the Jackson Rotary Club. He is also a member of Englewood Baptist Church and a grandfather of six.

Wishing Wall

There is a corridor at Le Bonheur Children's known as the Wishing Wall. Each person who wanders down this hallway is invited to make a wish, say a prayer, share a blessing or voice a hope. Pencils and half sheets of paper rest on pedestals for those who need them.

As chaplains, we have the rare privilege of reading the prayers, hopes, dreams and wishes written on those scraps of paper. We receive 20 to 30 wishes a day posted on that wall. Some of the wishes are silly or whimsical, such as "I want $86 million," or "I wish for a Mario Brothers video game," or "I want a pony." Some are expressions of heartfelt thanks for the staff's dedicated care and healing. Often, specific nurses, doctors and other staff members are mentioned by name, not only for their technical skills but also for their caring and compassionate hearts.

Other written secrets touch the very depth of our souls:

"I pray that my husband comes back home safe from the war, humble, and with the Lord deep within his soul."

"I pray we get a house."

"I pray that I could see my Dad."

"I hope to pass the sixth grade and for God to forgive me."

"Help my son be healed of ADHD and lose the generational curse off his life."

"I pray to stop them from garnishing my check and my daughter's check. We need money to pay bills. Please Lord, help me. Please!"

"Please pray for my mommy; they think she had a stroke."

"Prayers, wishes, hopes that the seizures go away, and I can become a marine biologist."

And simply, "I pray I am not sick anymore."

What ties these petitions together is heartfelt honesty and a longing for answers. Do not we all cast our longings outward when life is not as we expected? When we cry out for help, we are all the same. Rich or poor, black or white, healthy or sick, we are all the same in our need to be made whole.

We chaplains read over each of these wishes and then bring them to the Chapel, where we pray over them in union with their authors. Twice a week, the wishes are offered as prayers of petition to God during chapel services. Each month, some are included in the prayer offered before our hospital Town Hall meetings. At the end of each year, the sheets of paper are burned as a final offering, and the ashes are distributed to all who wish to receive them on Ash Wednesday.

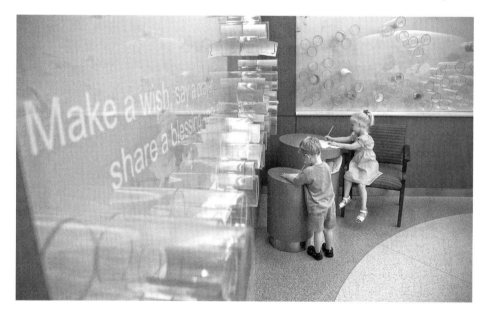

These petitions are rooted in the essence of who we are at Le Bonheur — an institution devoted to healing the body, mind and spirit of children. Le Bonheur is a special place where wishes, prayers, blessings and hopes never die.

Chaplain Jack Conrad is the manager of Le Bonheur's Spiritual Care team.

Soft Spot

L e Bonheur was born June 15, 1952, and I was born five days later. I've been here most of my life.

I came to Le Bonheur as an intern in 1978 after graduating from The University of Tennessee College of Medicine. Back then, the medical school had two classes each year. I graduated in December of 1977 and started at Le Bonheur the following January.

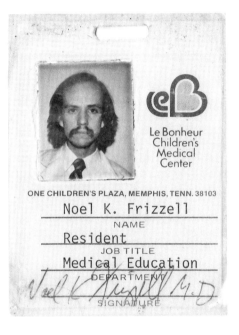

In 1978, we saw a tremendous number of infections due to the invasive H-flu disease. It caused a lot of very serious problems, and we dealt with infections ranging from meningitis to buccal cellulitis — all caused by the H-flu bacteria. Meningitis was the most severe, but we still saw it frequently. That year, we almost didn't go a single night on call without seeing some sort of serious H-flu infection.

I'd been working as an intern for about four months when I had a patient — a 4-month-old named Marcus — who had a serious H-flu infection. One of the complications of his infection was a subdural effusion, or collection of fluid beneath the dura covering his brain. Every day, I would go down to the infant care area on the ground floor of the hospital — known as the diarrhea dungeon — get a sterile tray and poke a needle into his soft spot to draw out the fluid. This kind of procedure was fairly common for us at that time.

Although his was a long and difficult infection, Marcus had a good outcome. I kept up with his progress after he recovered because his mother was on staff at Le Bonheur for many years. In my last update, I learned that Marcus is currently working on his master's degree.

I think the reason Marcus and his story mean so much to me is because it reminds me of the impact of vaccines in my lifetime. We have a vaccine for H-flu now, and we never see that type of serious infection anymore. Every day, I think about how much the practice of medicine has changed in the three decades that I've been doing this. In 1978, Le Bonheur was a little four-story community hospital. We didn't even have a CT scanner at that point; I remember having to transport kids over to another hospital just to get a scan. I also remember that, as an intern, I would work up a patient and then go back to the nursing station and light up a cigarette to chart my work. We had ashtrays at the nurses' stations and doctors who smoked on rounds. It was a totally different era.

Over the years, there have been remarkable changes not just with the medicine, but with the physical space. Le Bonheur's Central Tower opened up while I was a resident. In 2008, I watched the new hospital go up, and now I'm watching the Central Tower come down. I have watched Le Bonheur evolve from a community hospital to one of the nation's best institutions for caring for kids.

Dr. Noel "Kip" Frizzell has served as a Le Bonheur pediatrician for 34 years. In 1991, he founded Pediatric Consultants, and his practice is located in Le Bonheur's Outpatient Center.

Rising to the Occasion

E very day, the staff at Le Bonheur come to
work with the expectation that they will
provide care to help children heal, allowing
them to go about the business of growing up
among their families and friends. Sometimes
there are the days that challenge us to our
very core — the moments when we encounter
children who have been purposefully harmed,
traumatized and changed forever.

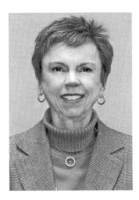

On March 3, 2008, six individuals — four adults and two
children — were killed during a home invasion in what is now known
as the "Lester Street" case. Three children survived the experience
but suffered severe injuries. These children were not discovered for
many hours and lay helpless in the home for almost a day, waiting
for rescue.

When these children were brought to Le Bonheur, it literally took
our breath away to see vulnerable little ones so tragically affected
by the most violent acts imaginable. They had experienced life-
altering physical attacks and required our most sophisticated medical
care. But the physical suffering was secondary to the effects of the
psychological trauma. Only hours earlier, these children had been
laughing and playing, enjoying an afternoon with their family and
friends. They came to us as orphans who had been brutally beaten,
existing in a morbid dream — not knowing where they were or whom
they could trust.

Our doctors and staff provided excellent medical care to
address the physical concerns, and the procedures went well. But as

challenging as it was to heal the physical wounds, our staff members were stretched to handle the psychological effects these children experienced as they began to emerge from the fog of anesthesia and medications. They were frightened and traumatized. They cried out for their parents, over and over again, inconsolably. They needed the security and comfort that only a loving family member could provide. But in the early hours of their recovery, we were not able to provide them with a family member because of the ongoing criminal investigation. This is where the Le Bonheur spirit truly emerged.

People at Le Bonheur rose to the occasion in two important ways. First, because the children did not have family available, Le Bonheur nurses and staff from several disciplines took shifts and assured that these children were held and rocked on a 24-hour basis as much as they needed. We had a constant flow of people who did everything possible to provide comfort and dry the tears. Secondly, we began coordinating with local officials to facilitate a reunion with loving grandparents and relatives — family members who were best able to calm the fears and bring some sense of normalcy to the children's shattered lives.

I was there the day that the children's grandmother walked into the Pediatric Intensive Care Unit and embraced these children for the first time since the incident. I saw the way they reached for her, held her close and clung to her for security and support. This was the first day that these children really began the healing process. Family made all the difference. And when family could not be there, Le Bonheur became their family.

Susan Steppe has worked at Le Bonheur for five years and served as the director of Social Work at the time of the Lester Street incident. She currently serves as project director of Community Integrated Services.

Snow Day

It was Valentine's Day 2008, and my son was undergoing surgery related to a tumor in his small intestine. We had been at Le Bonheur since Oct. 24 of the previous year.

It all began with a stomach ache that wouldn't go away. We'd been to see Jordan's pediatrician several times, who thought it was a case of lactose intolerance. We changed his diet, but Jordan didn't get better. And one day at school, he collapsed and began to vomit. We ended up at Le Bonheur.

Jordan went through a total of five surgeries. Although his tumor was benign, our surgeon, Dr. Max Langham, said it was one of the most difficult cases he had ever seen. Jordan stayed positive and never complained, but he was tired and didn't feel like doing much.

Then one afternoon, we had one of those rare March days in Memphis when it snowed, and there was really snow on the ground. I asked Jordan if he'd like to go outside and play in the snow. At first he said he didn't feel up to it. But after he looked outside the hospital room window and saw that the snow was sticking and still coming down, he agreed to go.

Outside the hospital, on the small lawn by Dunlap Street, I watched as my son enjoyed the falling snow. He had a big smile on his face — such a rarity those days — as he held out his tongue, capturing snowflakes. The sight of him so happy made me tear up. It was the first time he'd been outside since he was admitted to the hospital nearly six months ago.

We spent a total of 228 days in the hospital. Everyone — the doctors, nurses and other staff — was so friendly and made us feel like family. I decided that if I had to be anywhere other than home, it

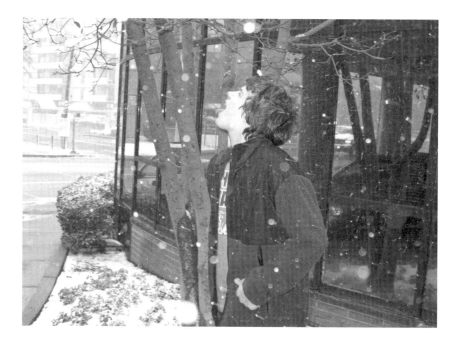

would be here at Le Bonheur. I'm grateful to Le Bonheur for helping my son. Not everyone gets to keep their child after an illness. 🩶

Jordan Hale is 18 years old and graduated from White Station High School in May 2012. His mother, Debbie Truska, says that he is completely healed and has figured out that girls like scars.

Ms. Flinn

Eulila Flinn joined the Le Bonheur laundry services department in 1955. She devoted the next 55 years of her life to the hospital. After spending some time in laundry services, she joined the Psychosocial Services team, where she delivered mail, packages and flowers, and escorted people where they needed to go.

I came to Le Bonheur in 1992, and by then, Ms. Flinn was already an institution around here. She loved kids so much, and she always

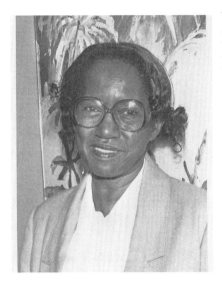

wanted to do for others. My first job here was working in the Emergency Department. Ms. Flinn and I often saw each other around the hospital, and she would always come by and speak to me. One day she overheard me say that I liked plain and simple cake, and after that, she made me a butter pound cake from scratch every Christmas. She'd bring it by and sneak it into my bottom drawer at work. They were so good.

Eventually, I started working in Psychosocial Services, and I loved working in the same department with Ms. Flinn. She was my good friend, and she did the work of many people. She accomplished so much during the day that, when she went on vacation, our team members would split her job between us just so we could do it right.

Ms. Flinn also ran the Le Bonheur clothes closet — a surplus of clothes, pajamas and other items for patients and families in need.

Ms. Flinn always knew exactly what we had and where to find the items, and she also knew what items were needed to help fill the closet. She would see kids in the lobby who didn't have socks on, and she would ask the families to wait, go to the clothes closet, pick out some socks and bring them back to the family. She'd tell the parents to make sure the kids had something on their feet, and they'd say, "Yes, ma'am."

Whenever people came to drop off clothing donations, Ms. Flinn lit up just like it was her personal closet. When Le Bonheur named the clothes closet after her, she had a happy fit. She was so humble; she never asked for anything or expected anything, and it was a really pleasant surprise for her.

In 2010, Ms. Flinn experienced some health problems and went out on sick leave. Even though she was on leave, every time I'd see her, she'd say, "How are my babies doing? I need to come back to Le Bonheur." Ms. Flinn passed away in the spring of 2011, and even now, people who were patients or parents of children here come by and ask about her. Sometimes they don't remember her name, but they always

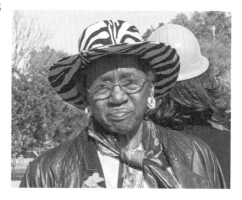

remember her by the words she said to everyone she encountered: "Thank God for another day and all His blessings."

Denise Norman has worked at Le Bonheur for 20 years, and she currently works as residency coordinator for the Neuroscience Institute.

Through the Bunny Room

My son, Jacob, is 12 years old. He has been hospitalized at Le Bonheur Children's 52 times since he was born. Eight of those hospital stays have included surgery.

Until June 18, 2009, few parents at Le Bonheur ever accompanied their child back to the Operating Room for surgery, and that was always for special circumstances. The Family Partners Council, a group of parent advisers at the hospital, had been talking for awhile about how we wanted to go back with our children for induction before surgery. We were working with the team at Le Bonheur to see about making our dream a reality.

The reason the Family Partners are so adamant about being able to go back when our children go for induction is because we have parents on the council whose children never came out of surgery. And it's hard on children and parents when the child is taken away. We've all talked about having our child reach out to us crying, "No Mommy, don't let them take me." After Jacob goes back, I always wonder, "What's happening to him? Is it cold? Is someone comforting him?"

Jacob was scheduled to have tendon release surgery for his club foot, and his anesthesiologist, Dr. Poorna Subramaniam, had come to Le Bonheur from a hospital where parents went back for induction. Dr. Jeff Sawyer, Jacob's orthopedic surgeon, was also on board with the idea, and we decided to try it. I would be the first parent at Le Bonheur to accompany a child to the OR.

The day came for Jacob's surgery, and I dressed out in a bunny suit. Our plan was that I would carry him back, hold his hand and, once he was asleep, I would leave. I picked up my son, and we walked

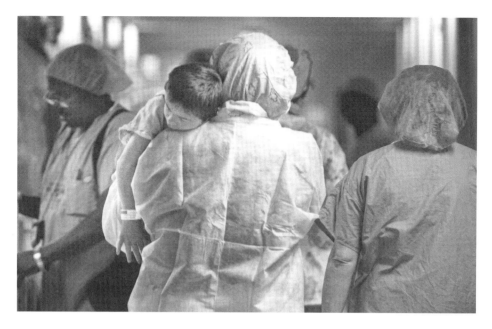

together through the Bunny Room.

When we crossed the threshold into the OR, it was amazing how everything changed. The lighting was different — more intense — there was an antiseptic smell, and there was a temperature change. The temperature dropped. I hadn't expected that — that it would feel so different. Even the sound was different because of the hard tile, it almost seemed like there was a bit of an echo as we walked down that hallway.

We walked into the OR suite, and Dr. Poorna told me to lay Jacob down on the table. It was surprisingly warm; there was some sort of warming blanket on the table, and that alleviated my first fear. He wasn't just lying on a cold table.

It was very quiet in the OR. People to my left were preparing the instruments, and Dr. Sawyer was standing beside me. Dr. Poorna told me to hold Jacob's hand and asked me if I wanted to sing to him, and then she put the mask on and told Jacob she was using the cherry scent we had picked. I was surprised at how quickly he went to sleep.

I felt his hand go limp, and then Dr. Poorna told me they had him from here. She was so gentle with him. She had the mask on his face, but she was also rubbing his cheek. That was another fear alleviated. I knew that Jacob wasn't just an object — that the people in the room truly cared about him.

I don't remember who took my hand and walked me out, but I remember feeling so relieved, having gone back with him. Knowing that it wasn't scary for him. And I realized I was very comfortable with the whole process.

Joanne Cunningham is the director of patient- and family-centered care for Methodist Le Bonheur Healthcare, and she served as the first chairperson for Le Bonheur's Family Partners Council.

Relaxin'

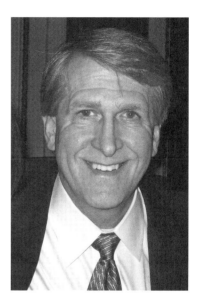

In 1977, I was a first-year medical student working as a suture tech in the Emergency Department at Le Bonheur. One day, two young brothers — Jerome and El Paso — presented to the ED with cuts. Jerome, the 5-year-old, had a cut on his finger, and El Paso, 3 years old, had a cut on his chin.

Both boys required stitches, and big brother Jerome went first. I stitched up his finger and prepared to fix up El Paso as well. When it came to El Paso's turn, he was pitching a fit and didn't want me to come near him. We had to restrain him so that I could safely stitch up his chin, and his screams let everyone — including Jerome — know how upset he was.

As soon as I got to work on El Paso's chin, Jerome ran up behind me and started hitting me, yelling, "Let my brother loose! Let him go!" I turned to Jerome and explained that I needed to fix El Paso's chin, and I told Jerome to have a seat on the chair behind the exam table and relax.

By this time, El Paso had completely worn himself out and was fast asleep. He slept soundly while I gave him stitches, and we finished up without incident.

When I turned around to check on Jerome, I saw that he was doing exactly as he was told — calmly sitting in the chair behind the exam table. I noticed, though, that there was one empty bottle of sterile water on the table and a second bottle in Jerome's hand. Between his fingers, Jerome was holding a green ink pen.

Surprised, I asked him, "Jerome, what are you doing with that water and pen?" He looked at me and replied, "Well, I'm relaxin' — drinking a beer and smoking a cigarette."

Dr. Lelon Edwards — better known around town as Dr. Bubba — graduated from The University of Tennessee College of Medicine, completed his residency at Le Bonheur and worked as a physician in Le Bonheur's Emergency Department for four years. He has been in practice at Pediatrics East since 1988.

True Friends

In 1998, we spent nearly two months at Le Bonheur with my 11-year-old son, David Paul. My son was brought to the hospital on Feb. 13 after he was accidentally shot with a hunting rifle by one of his friends. He was flown by helicopter from Savannah, Tenn., to The Regional Medical Center before he was taken to Le Bonheur. The accident caused severe damage to his pelvis, spinal cord and intestines, and he underwent more than one surgery at Le Bonheur. The nurses and staff were so kind and caring during that entire time. They cared not only for David Paul, but for my family and me, too.

One of David Paul's favorite nurses, Sherry McNabb, gave him extra special treatment. One night, when David Paul's feeding tube was removed, Sherry drove all over Memphis to find his favorite dessert — Sara Lee cherry cheesecake. She finally found a store that was open after hours and carried that kind of cheesecake. She brought it back to David Paul, who was so excited to eat his favorite treat.

When David Paul was finally discharged in late April, Sherry drove home with us even though it was her day off. David Paul was brought home by ambulance, and, because I get car sick,

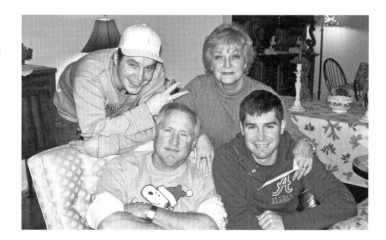

I had to sit in the front with the driver. Sherry sat in the back with David Paul, so he wouldn't feel alone or scared.

Sherry wasn't the only one to go above and beyond to make David Paul feel better during his stay. One day when David Paul went down for an X-ray, he complimented the technician's Winnie the Pooh tie. The technician immediately whipped it off and gave it to David Paul. Even though we protested, he insisted, saying it "looked better on David Paul." We still have that tie.

And one of the Food Services staff members noted that many times the only thing missing off David Paul's food tray was his blue Jell-o. His appetite was slow to return, but from that day forward, there was always blue Jell-o on David's tray. She also encouraged me to eat when she noticed the weight I was losing from stress.

Hospital staff even allowed David's best friend from school to spend spring break camped out on a cot in his room. They did physical therapy together, played bingo on the house TV and entertained each other despite the agonizing pain David was in.

Everyone at Le Bonheur was always concerned about all of us, not just David Paul. They cared for us as a family, knowing we all needed healing. When the weight of the ordeal seemed more than I could carry, there was always someone there willing to share the load — an act only a true friend can offer.

Paula Dotson lives in Sheffield, Ala., with her husband, David, and their two sons, David Paul — top left — and Bradley. David Paul has limited feeling below the waist but has learned to walk, drive a car and do many other things through the use of his big toes.

Sunshine Girls

In the early years at Le Bonheur, the ladies of Le Bonheur Club did all sorts of jobs at the hospital. Members hosted a tea room with drinks and sandwiches, staffed a wonderful hospital library filled with all the books you'd find in any public library and took carts of books around twice a day to every child in the hospital. We also ran the elevators; people would get on and tell us what floor, and then we would push the buttons and take them where they needed to go. My very first day running the elevators, I was wearing a bright yellow uniform, and I was so nervous because I had quite a fear of getting stuck in elevators. Dr. Jimmy Hughes got in that elevator and rode up and down with me for 30 minutes, so I'd feel more relaxed. Another time, Dr. Don Winfield rode around with me for a long while telling jokes and keeping me company.

Club members manned the front desk, worked in the gift shop, sorted and delivered the mail and worked in the sewing room.

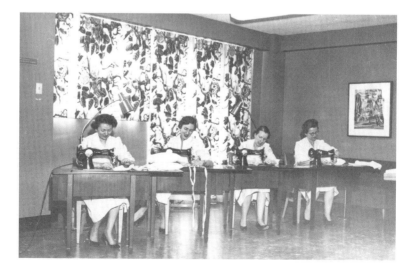

We also had a group called the Sunshine Girls who would sit in rooms with the children, read to them and keep them company. When Le Bonheur first opened, members worked 48 three-hour shifts a year — about one shift a week — and they kept us hopping. If you finished your shift before three hours, then you went on to another job.

Many of our shifts were spent in the sewing room. The club made every piece of clothing that was used in the hospital — gowns for the children, uniforms for the nurses, surgical gowns for the physicians, doctors' masks, sheets for the beds and even toys for the Bunny Room. There weren't any throwaways back then. Mrs. Irene Schaeffer ruled the sewing room with an iron hand. She was an institution. Irene taught a lot of people to sew, if you can believe that. Many women who had never sewn before went up there to do shifts, so Irene would show them how to make whatever they were working on. You got to know the other members well while sewing together, and you learned everything that was going on with people we knew.

No matter what your job was, you didn't miss a shift. Le Bonheur and the other club members counted on you to be there, and you didn't just call in and say you weren't coming. One morning before a shift, I realized I had a flat tire, so I called a cab in order to get to the hospital on time. You just didn't miss your turn to do something worthwhile for Le Bonheur. 🤍

Le Bonheur Club is a non-profit organization supporting Le Bonheur Children's Hospital through fundraising and volunteer service. Club members Bette Lathram, Billie Anne Williams, Ann Whitsett, Gloria Andereck, Sue Cheek Hughes, Elaine Colmer and Anita Pharr contributed their memories to this story.

Bucket List

In 2007, I wrote a story on Le Bonheur's nephrology program for *Le Bonheur* magazine. We needed a patient to feature on the cover, and when I talked to our nephrology team about a good candidate, everyone agreed that the patient whose spirit captured the true face of Le Bonheur's dialysis unit was Jermaine Chamberlain.

In June, I met Jermaine during one of his three-times-a-week dialysis treatments. Until then, all the stories I had written for the hospital's magazine were about very young children, and I had interviewed their parents. Jermaine was 16, and hearing his story told in his own words made for a remarkable and truly memorable interview.

Jermaine was so positive, cheerful, upbeat and optimistic — a joyful youth and a delight to be around. He was funny, charming, friendly and outgoing, and we hit it off immediately.

Jermaine was born with kidney disease and began dialysis when he was 2 days old, under the care of Le Bonheur's nephrology physicians. As an infant, he was removed from the home of his biological family and placed in custodial care. During the search to find him a foster family, he was "adopted" by Le Bonheur's dialysis team, and for the first 21 months of his life, he lived at the hospital. The staff in the Dialysis Unit cared for him, bought him clothes and treated him like their own child until wonderful foster parents — Linda and Tony Chamberlain — took Jermaine in and then adopted him into their family.

In October, after his story was published, I took Jermaine copies of the magazine with his big, bright smile beaming from the cover. He was so proud and autographed copies for his friends.

When I learned Jermaine's story had garnered the top feature writing award in a national competition, I couldn't wait to tell him. I knew he would be very proud to learn that his story had made such an impact on so many others throughout the country. He shared my joy. Two months later, he shared his story again on the radio during Le Bonheur's annual radiothon.

Jermaine turned 21 on Nov. 11, 2011, and graduated from Le Bonheur's Dialysis Unit to an adult dialysis center on Nov. 30. By then we had become friends, and I thought I'd probably never see him again. It was one of the most tearful days of my life.

But since leaving Le Bonheur, Jermaine continues to visit the Dialysis Unit and is an incredible role model for other dialysis patients. He also visits me from time to time.

When Jermaine stopped by my office in March, I had recently read that the Memphis Zoo was offering camel rides as a special attraction. I asked if he had ever wanted to ride a camel. I told him riding a camel was on my bucket list, and I asked him to join me. He loved the idea.

On April 10, we went to the Memphis Zoo, rode a camel named Mickey and saw every exhibit.

Afterward, we went out for hamburgers. Over dinner, I asked Jermaine what he tells other dialysis patients who struggle with their disease. He said, "I tell them I'm grateful I have kidney disease."

I was stunned and asked him what he meant.

Jermaine said, "Some things that are really horrible can become a blessing. If I didn't have kidney disease, I wouldn't have been surrounded by people from all walks of life who have showered me with love and affection. If it weren't for Le Bonheur, I wouldn't have accomplished all the things that I always wanted to do."

He told me he had always wanted to be on TV, the radio, in the newspaper and in a magazine, and because of Le Bonheur, he had done all of those things.

I was incredibly moved by his words. Then it struck me — Jermaine had started his bucket list years ago. I laughed and told him I had some catching up to do!

Jermaine has been an inspiring influence, and knowing him has truly changed my life. As we plan our next bucket list adventure, I can't help but reflect that if it weren't for Le Bonheur, our bucket lists would never have started. Jermaine will always be my inspiration to remain forever young and enjoy every day to the fullest.

Kini Kedigh Plumlee has worked in communications at Le Bonheur for seven years and is the editor of Le Bonheur *magazine. Jermaine Chamberlain is 21 years old, and he and Kini are currently planning their next bucket list adventure. To honor Jermaine and the caregivers on Le Bonheur's dialysis unit, Kini has made a planned gift to Le Bonheur's nephrology research fund.*

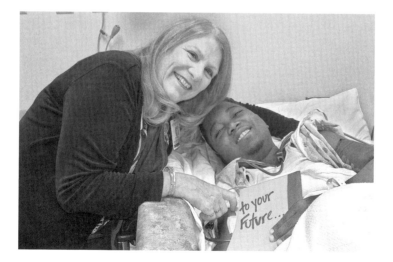

Happy Tears

M y daughter, Caitlyn, was born with cloacal exstrophy — a
condition in which much of the abdominal organs, including
the bladder and the intestines, are present outside of the body. I
work as a nurse at Le Bonheur, and Caitlyn recently had an 11-hour
operation here to help correct her condition. Several months ago, we
had an appointment with Radiology to take a scan of Caitlyn's hips
in preparation for the surgery. During the appointment, our MRI
tech, Becky Weidner, was wonderful — very informative and caring.

A few weeks after Caitlyn's MRI, I was sitting at my desk and
received a phone call from Becky. She couldn't give me much
information due to patient privacy laws, but Becky told me a mother
and infant were currently in Radiology. The infant had bladder
exstrophy, and the mother had expressed a desire to meet another
family in the area with the same condition. Without providing any
further details, Becky asked me if I was interested in coming down to
meet the mother, and I went downstairs right away.

When I got to the waiting area near MRI/CT, I found Becky,
and she walked me over to the mother. The mother looked confused
because I was wearing my operating room scrubs and hat. Then Becky
said, "This is Bre, and she is the mother of Caitlyn, who has bladder
exstrophy." Immediately, the mother, Adrienne, and I started hugging
and crying. I learned that her daughter, Anna Grace, is only three
weeks older than Caitlyn. Becky showed us to a private area where we
could talk and cry happy tears together.

Having a child diagnosed with a major defect is extremely scary,
and any support a person or family can find is a true blessing. Becky

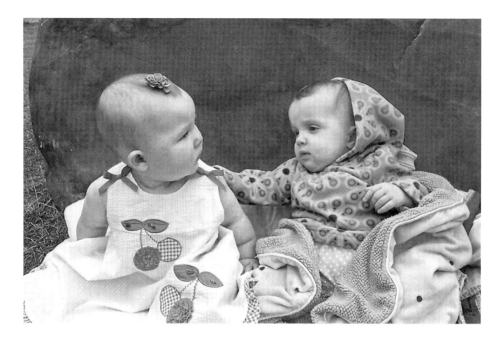

recognized this need in both of us during separate visits, and without pushing or divulging protected information, she was able to bring us together. Both of our daughters are going through the same major ordeal, and Adrienne and I talk with each other daily. We've helped each other cope and feel more normal. I can't tell Becky enough how much I appreciate what she has done for our families. We know we and our daughters will be lifelong friends, and I know God put Becky in our path for this very reason. 💛

Breanne Curry works as a clinical educator for Perioperative Services at Le Bonheur. Previously, she served as a patient care coordinator in the hospital's OR. Adrienne Furr-McTyre is now a member of the Methodist Le Bonheur Healthcare Family Partners Council. Her daughter, Anna Grace, often has play dates with Caitlyn.

I Might Last a Week

Ibegan working in the Operating Room at Le Bonheur in 1976. I was stationed at the front desk and did a variety of jobs — everything from scheduling surgeries and running blood gases to answering pagers and phones for surgeons while they were operating.

On my very first day of work, heart surgeon Dr. Robert "Bobby" Allen came over to my desk, took off his bloody gloves and threw

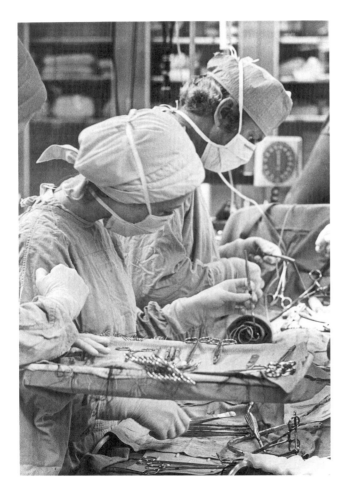

them on the desk. My father was a therapist, so I considered myself familiar with the medical field. But after Dr. Allen threw those gloves down, I thought, "OK. I might last a week."

We had a very small OR at that time. There were three general surgeons on staff — Drs. Robert Hollabaugh, Earle Wrenn and Bobby Allen.

Dr. Doug Hixson was a resident. Back then, we ran only six operating rooms. We had a manual typewriter and a mimeograph machine, and I would type up the next day's schedule each afternoon and run off copies on the mimeograph machine in Admissions. The intercom system was interesting, too. It was a little 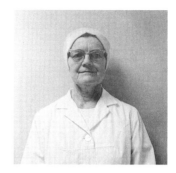 box that transmitted only to the doctors' lounge and the nurses' lounge. We had to flip the switch down to talk and lift it up to hear. We'd use it to let the doctors know their patients had arrived.

Mrs. Alice Cantrell supervised the OR. She was strict, but she ran an excellent OR. She would never let us address one another by our first names. It was always Miss, Ms. or Mrs. No one was allowed into the nurses' station — where I sat — except Mrs. Cantrell and me. Even the doctors weren't allowed to come in and use the phone. Dr. Allen always threatened to install a pay phone in the OR.

Dr. Allen was a real character. He always wore a headlight to operate, and I remember once, he was fussing because the nurse couldn't get his headlight to stay in place. Frustrated because it was crooked, he said, "There's nothing wrong with this light. It's not lopsided," and the nurse said, "No, sir, but your ears are." In all my time at Le Bonheur, we only shut down the OR once, and that was when Dr. Allen died in a car wreck. We closed down the entire OR so everyone could attend the funeral.

The strangest phone call I ever took was once when a resident's wife called while he was in surgery. She was in tears at their vet's office, and I had to walk into the OR and ask her husband what antibiotic she needed to tell the vet to prescribe for their pet turtle. He gave me a name, and I came back out and told the vet. I never found out if the turtle survived.

One year — around the time the movie E.T. came out — our department entered the hospital-wide Christmas decorating contest. In the spirit of E.T., we went with an "Out of this World Christmas" theme. We decorated the nurses' station in aluminum foil and had flashing lights everywhere. The nurses made an E.T. character out of paper mache. We won the contest that year.

The OR was a good place to work. I first came to Le Bonheur to fill in for a friend for six weeks while she had an operation. Then in December of that year, the hospital called and asked if I would be interested in working full time. I came for the interview and loved the people, so I took the job, and I've been here ever since. I love the kids. Le Bonheur has been wonderful to me and for me.

Bennie Haynes has worked at Le Bonheur since 1976. She currently serves as a Quality Improvement specialist.

Something to Give

I've worked at Le Bonheur for 12 years, and for the past eight years, I've served as coordinator of our Brain Tumor Program. My greatest inspiration is watching our families and staff pull together time after time, creating a team approach to patient care in the face of a devastating diagnosis.

One patient who stands out in my mind came to Le Bonheur in 2009 for treatment of a highly malignant brain tumor. Her other caregivers and I quickly realized there was something special about this girl — a strong sense of selflessness, courage, beauty and compassion, even though she was battling for her life. She never complained, and whenever she got a toy, she would give it away to another child. She was always so concerned for everyone else.

This patient was at Le Bonheur several times throughout the course of her disease. She underwent a few surgeries on her tumor and required hospitalization at other times as well. As we came toward the end and knew we wouldn't be able to save her, our focus became more about her quality of life.

At one point, the family was supposed to go on a Make-A-Wish trip to Hawaii, but the girl became very sick, and her trip was postponed. She was very depressed. To cheer her up, our staff decorated her room like a luau, and we had a party for days. We ate Hawaiian food and hung decorations and everyone wore leis on the unit, and she could not stop smiling. Eventually she did get to travel to Hawaii, and she used her spending money to buy gifts for staff and friends on the unit. As caregivers, she taught us what it means to be selfless and that no matter what you're facing, you always have something to give.

As things progressed with her disease, this child became distressed that she might not see her two little dogs again. She loved those dogs, and at home, they stayed by her side constantly. We partnered with Child Life and made arrangements, and her two dogs were able to come and stay with her here in the hospital. The moment we brought the animals in the room, I saw peace come across her face. Her parents were so relieved. They told me that we had done the best thing possible for their daughter — more than medicine or surgery could do. Sometimes she felt well enough to go out in the garden with her dogs, and they stayed with her through the end of her life.

This girl's family still stays very connected to Le Bonheur, and they have established a closet on the neuroscience floor in her memory. The closet is fully stocked with toys, games and other activities to give to inpatients on the unit. Even though their daughter is in heaven, she's still touching lives every day.

Tracy Tidwell has worked at Le Bonheur for 12 years. She currently serves as Brain Tumor Program director.

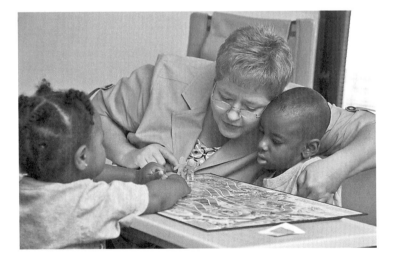

The Right Decision

I've been on staff at Le Bonheur since 1982. In the past three decades, I've seen significant advances in the field of pediatric medicine – both in our understanding of disease processes and in the level of care we are able to provide to patients. Today, I'm treating kids whose parents were patients of mine when they were children. The parents 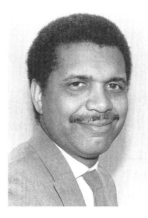 sometimes relate events to me that I don't recall, but they remember. They talk about how they appreciated the care they received when they were kids. Sometimes, a parent I cared for won't recognize me, but then the child's grandmother might come in and say, "Well, you know he took care of you when you were admitted to Le Bonheur and you were sick." It makes me think that we did a good job, to have a family remember us fondly many years later.

For a number of years, I cared for a young lady who had received a heart transplant. I was her general pediatrician, so I coordinated between the cardiologist, the transplant surgeon and a number of other providers. The child's family lived in Blytheville, but they came to Le Bonheur because they felt they would receive the best care here. During the course of the child's treatment, I began to feel like I was a family member. I knew the family, they trusted my judgment and they considered my opinion on many of the issues that arose concerning the patient.

When you are the recipient of a transplant organ, you are placed on immunosuppressive agents. And with those drugs, there is a higher chance of developing a malignancy, or cancer. Eventually, this child developed a malignant tumor. Her family knew that if they stopped the immunosuppressive agents, the cancer would regress, but her heart would fail. Another option was to continue the agents and administer chemotherapy, which of course also has adverse side effects. At the peak of this patient's illness, the family was faced with this difficult decision.

The child was in Le Bonheur's Intensive Care Unit and there was a huge team gathered — family, extended family, the transplant team, oncologists, someone from the ethics committee — and all of the options were laid out. Ultimately, the family decided to take their daughter home and not put her through any more treatment. After they made that decision, everyone left, but the family asked me to stay. They asked me if I thought they were making the right choice. I agreed with them. In situations like theirs, you have to think in terms of suffering and quality of life — and to me, that's what the family was thinking about. They felt like enough was enough, and they were right. The young lady died within a week, and she was able to die at home, surrounded by her family.

I still occasionally get a card from them or messages from the family through one of the cardiac coordinators, even though this was at least 15 years ago. It was rewarding to provide care to a very special child and to be considered a family member. Some very difficult decisions had to be made at the end, and I felt honored to provide support and help the family make what they felt was the right decision.

The reason I stay and continue to do what I do is twofold. One, Le Bonheur is a teaching institution, so I'm truly affecting people who will practice medicine for the next 20, 30 and 40 years. I hope that I can mentor our students and residents and serve as an example of the type of physician they should become. And two, being based at Le Bonheur allows me not to think about a family's financial ability. I can focus on the patient and provide the best care for their disease. That's why I choose to stay here. Interacting with medical students, residents, and the patients and their families makes it worthwhile.

Gerald Presbury moved to Memphis in 1982 for a fellowship in hematology/ oncology at St. Jude Children's Research Hospital. He has treated patients at Le Bonheur for the past 30 years and is currently a member of UT/ Le Bonheur Pediatric Specialists.

BASH Unit

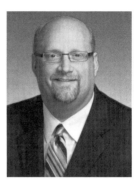

My first encounter with Le Bonheur was in 1994. My wife and I were expecting our third child and learned that she would be born with spina bifida. At the time, we were living in Trenton, Tenn., with our two young sons, Bill and Jonathan. We did some research, and Le Bonheur neurosurgeon Dr. Robert Sanford came up as one of the top physicians in the country for treating spina bifida. I called Dr. Sanford, and he invited us to come to Memphis and take a tour of Le Bonheur. My wife and I went to meet with him, and he talked us through everything we were facing. Then, we toured the hospital, and the staff discussed how our daughter would be transported, her plan of care and other key details. We also conducted phone interviews with doctors in New Orleans and Chicago, but we decided that Le Bonheur was the right place for us.

A few months after our tour, Mary Kathryn was born. I spent the first 10 days of her life sleeping on the floor in her room. The clinical care was excellent, but I was blown away by the people. From the Environmental Services workers and the nurses who fussed at me if I didn't wash my hands to Mr. Clint Trusty — a volunteer who came to rock babies who didn't have family members around — and the folks in the cafeteria, it was obvious how much everyone loved these kids.

When it was time to go home, I left Le Bonheur thankful for what they did for Mary Kathryn, but I also left thinking that this was the kind of place where I wanted to work. At that point in my career I was a salesman, but six months later, I got a job working for the

Le Bonheur Foundation.

My first role in development was to create a regional fundraising program designed to raise awareness of Le Bonheur outside of Memphis. I designed a float called the BASH Unit — the Bear Ambulatory Surgical Hospital — and filled it with stuffed animals, as well as my own children. I pulled the float in four parades throughout West Tennessee in an effort to put Le Bonheur on people's minds. It was the goofiest looking float, but it worked. When people saw the BASH Unit, they would call and ask me to come speak to their clubs and organizations.

I also worked a great deal with Walmart, Dairy Queen and other Children's Miracle Network partners. At one point, I was asked to call on Walmart and encourage them to increase their giving. One store requested that, if they increased their giving by 25 percent, I would do something silly to motivate their staff. I agreed, and when they reached their goal, they asked me to dress up as a woman and work as a greeter for an afternoon. So, for four hours, I wore a dress and a wig and greeted customers at the Walmart Supercenter in Jackson, Tenn. We did everything we could think of to raise money for Le Bonheur.

Eventually, I became involved in the hospital's advocacy and government relations division. When I left Le Bonheur, I served as the director of the Tennessee governor's office of Children's Care Coordination. All of the work I have done in children's health care for the past 18 years is because of Le Bonheur, and I am forever grateful and indebted to the hospital for having that impact on me.

Bob Duncan currently serves as executive vice president at Children's Hospital of Wisconsin. He and his wife, Sarah, live in Sussex, Wis., with Mary Kathryn, who is 18 years old.

Baby Food on Toast

The closest thing to my heart, I guess, is Le Bonheur. It was my life. It's a place where sick children are — and always have been — welcome.

I wanted to be a pediatrician ever since I was a Boy Scout. I knew there was no way I could do anything but take care of children. Nothing can make you feel more special than saving a baby's life.

I got my first taste of being a doctor when I worked as a hospital corpsman on a Navy ship during World War II. After boot camp and medical corpsman training, I spent four years treating soldiers for colds, ear infections and the occasional appendicitis.

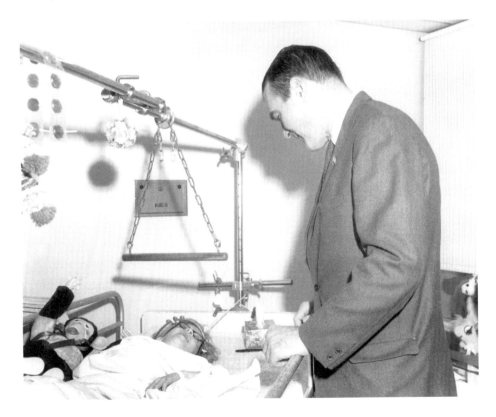

Of everything I've accomplished in life, I am most proud of being Le Bonheur's first resident physician in the mid-1950s. I trained at The University of Tennessee and then completed my internship at the John Gaston Hospital. Dr. Ray Paul and I performed the first heart catheterizations on children in Memphis.

I ate a lot of baby food on toast in the middle of the night at Le Bonheur. I had a bed upstairs in the tower, and I lived there, really. It was my life. I remember crying with parents, talking to moms and learning what they worry about.

What I've learned about children is that they know immediately whether you love them. Well into my 80s, I could hardly wait to get back to my clinic on Monday mornings to see the kids. I think my experience helped calm upset mothers who are still learning how to raise babies.

Emmett Bell Jr. was a physician at Memphis Children's Clinic until retiring in 2011. He served as Le Bonheur's first resident physician in the mid-1950s.

Like Family

In March of 2006, our 10-month-old daughter, Madeline, began to have episodes where, when she cried really hard, she would pass out for a few seconds. It almost looked like she was falling asleep for a moment. In the course of a few days, it happened a handful of times, and then on a Sunday, she experienced two episodes — once on a walk when a dog startled her and another at home when she toppled over while leaning against a chair. My husband, Tim, and I called our pediatrician's office and made an appointment for Monday morning. After Madeline passed out at the doctor's office for almost 20 seconds, an ambulance was called to take us to Le Bonheur.

From the Le Bonheur Emergency Department, our daughter was admitted to the hospital and underwent a battery of tests, which indicated that something was wrong with her heart. On our fourth day at Le Bonheur, she had an appointment in the Cath Lab to determine exactly what was wrong. Tim and I sat in the waiting room in the Intensive Care Unit late into the evening waiting to receive the news. Finally, Drs. Glenn Wetzel and Joel Lutterman — Le Bonheur cardiologists — came to give us the results. We learned that our baby had an atrial septal defect — a congenital heart condition — as well

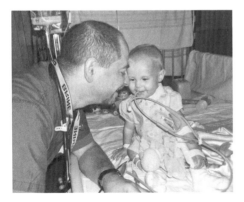

as an arrhythmia, a cleft in her mitral valve and pulmonary hypertension. The defects would require surgery, and if the only medicine currently available to treat her hypertension didn't work, there would be nothing else they could do. It was a devastating diagnosis.

When the doctors left, it was nearly midnight. I went down to Le Bonheur's lactation room to pump milk for Madeline. It was an incredibly emotional moment for me, bottling milk for my little girl after hearing everything she was about to face. On my way back upstairs, Dr. Lutterman was walking out of the elevator. He saw me standing there, bottles in my hands and tears in my eyes, and he hugged me and said, "We're going to get through this. Are you OK?" He told me Madeline's care team would talk through our options and work things out. At that point, I had only known him for two days, and I was moved and comforted by his gesture and his words of encouragement. He was real, but he was optimistic.

Madeline had surgery a week later, and Dr. Lutterman continued to be reassuring. He drew pictures of Madeline's heart on exam table paper to help us understand cardiac anatomy, and he combined patience with a comfortable sense of humor. He gave me his e-mail address and cell phone number, letting us know we could contact him at any time. We knew we had a friend in Dr. Joel. During the next few years, Madeline underwent more heart caths and more surgeries, but Le Bonheur helped us through it.

Madeline continues to get check-ups regularly, and we still keep in touch with Dr. Joel. On Doctors' Day this year, we texted him a recording of our children singing him a silly song. The care he provided for Madeline will always be appreciated, and we update him on her progress like a member of our family. That's what Le Bonheur is to us — a family.

Bridgette and Tim Flack both serve on Le Bonheur's Family Partners Council, and Bridgette also volunteers as a parent mentor in the hospital's Cardiovascular Intensive Care Unit. They live in Memphis, Tenn., with their three children — Madeline, 7, Eli, 4, and Susanna, 2.

Medical Mission

On Jan. 12, 2010, an earthquake shook the capital city of Haiti, killing more than 200,000 people and leaving massive devastation in its wake. The U.S. government contacted the National Association of Children's Hospitals and Related Institutions seeking help from pediatric specialists to provide aid in Haiti. Le Bonheur volunteered to send a 10-person surgical trauma team to Port-au-Prince.

Before coming to Le Bonheur, I worked as a paramedic and responded to many natural disasters. Because of my past experience, I was asked to advise the team on supplies and logistics for the medical mission to Haiti. One of the worst things that you can do in a disaster is to come unprepared. I wanted to make sure our team was fully equipped for every possible scenario, so that we would be helpful, not hurtful.

Our supply list quickly grew from a few items to enough medical resources to fill two 40-foot trailers. Thankfully, FedEx had offered to fly over our team and supplies at no cost. Drawing from my administrative experience in Le Bonheur's Emergency Department, I thought about the number of patients we might see each day and the supplies we would need to treat common injuries and illnesses. Items ranged from bandages and medications to surgical equipment and a rabies vaccination kit.

One week before the team departed, I was asked to join the mission and travel with them to Haiti. I had packed the supplies and knew what we had, where it was and how to use it. Luckily, we were so busy preparing for departure that I didn't have much idle time to worry about the trip. I used my experience as a paramedic to help mentally prepare myself for the devastation we would face.

After we arrived in Haiti and our supplies were unloaded and organized, I shifted gears and returned to my roots as a paramedic. The trip provided me with an opportunity to step away from administrative challenges and just take care of people all day. The people we took care of were so grateful. They would stand in line for hours to be seen by a doctor, and they were always smiling and thankful.

My most memorable patient in Haiti was a middle-aged man

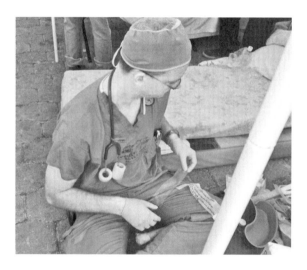

named Michael. Like most Haitians, Michael performed hard physical labor to provide for his family. In the earthquake, he sustained a femur fracture and developed a severe infection in his leg. Dr. Sunny Anand and I cared for Michael for eight days trying to fight the infection, but it wasn't getting better. On our last day at Sacred Heart Hospital, it was clear that amputation was the only hope of saving Michael's life. He would either lose his leg or he would die.

I went into the tent to check on Michael, and he pleaded with me, asking what else I could do to heal him. He couldn't lose his leg and still provide for his family. My most difficult moment was looking him in the eye and telling him that we'd done all we could do and this was his only option. There was a sense of failure that we'd worked so hard to heal the infection, and it wouldn't heal. I have tremendous respect for Michael for fighting to provide for his family, and I hate that I couldn't give him the happy ending he wanted. I hope he has been able to find a new life with a prosthetic.

We did experience many success stories — rewarding moments helping people to walk again, to get up and work through their pain, to reach a point where they had a better chance of going home. When I worked as a paramedic before, I never got to see my patients get better. In Haiti, the best part was seeing my patients improve and heal. It reinforced why I went into medicine.

Since we've returned to Memphis and Le Bonheur, I think of our time in Haiti and remember why I love what I do. All people deserve to be cared for. Medicine is a calling, and it isn't easy, but it is an opportunity to make someone's life better.

S. Crile Crisler has worked at Le Bonheur Children's since 2004. He currently serves as administrative director of Emergency Services.

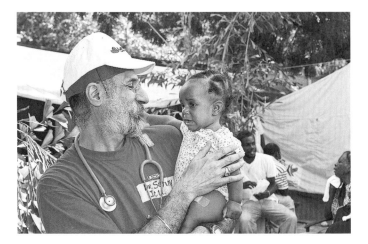

Courage and Lucky

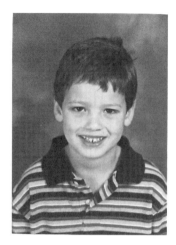

I n 2002, our son, Brendan, was 7 years old and a student at Chimneyrock Elementary. One afternoon, our neighbor, who was picking Brendan up from school, called and said there had been an accident at the school. As soon as I got there, I knew things were more serious than I realized. I saw helicopters and ambulances, but I still didn't know just how bad the situation was. I ran up to the carpool line and saw Brendan lying face down on the pavement. He was one of nine kids who had been hit by a car that drove through a group of kids waiting in the carpool line. Brendan was airlifted to Le Bonheur with severe head injuries, broken bones and lots of abrasions.

We weren't sure Brendan would make it through that first night, and for the next several days, we had no idea of his prognosis. There was a long path of unknowns, and the doctors couldn't be sure if he would be paralyzed or whether he would ever see or hear again.

One memory of our stay remains very vivid in my mind. The first night we spent in the Pediatric Intensive Care Unit, I was sitting at Brendan's bedside with Dr. Mark Bugnitz. He was telling me stories about Christmas lights. He talked about how his neighbors try to outdo one another each year and his plan for his own lights. I was still in a state of shock, but I listened. I didn't realize it at the time, but now I see the kindness and caring behind his gesture as he tried to distract me. One of the hardest things to do in such a dire situation is wait and hope for the best. Dr. Bugnitz was doing what he could to take my mind somewhere else.

A few days later, one of the PICU nurses brought Brendan two Beanie Babies — a kind gesture that, unbeknownst to us, would become our symbol of hope and healing. One was white and covered with green clovers. His name was Lucky. The other was red, white and blue and named Courage. Those Beanie Babies went with Brendan everywhere, even though he didn't know they were there. They were with him for every test, procedure and surgery. They were by his side at all times.

It wasn't until the 10th day of our stay that Brendan began to wake up. We still weren't sure of the extent of his injuries, especially to his brain, and what permanent damage would remain. We waited patiently as he opened his eyes. We cried and told him how much we loved him; we tried to explain where he was and what was happening. He looked around at all of the tubes and machines and promptly picked up one of the Beanie Babies and threw it in frustration. That's when we began to breathe again. That's when we knew Brendan was going to be OK. Ten years later, those Beanie Babies are still with us. They serve as a symbol of hope and remind us of the moment we knew our son would heal. 💚

Karen Eskin lives in Germantown, Tenn., with her husband, Marc, and their three children. Brendan is 16 and a sophomore at Houston High School. He runs cross country and track.

It's Alive!

In the summer of 1974, my husband, Michael, took a job as general manager for the Minnesota Vikings. The job required him to move to Minnesota almost immediately, so I stayed behind in Memphis with our 5-year-old son, Mike, to pack up the house and make preparations to join him.

It was an August day not long after Michael had moved, and I was at home packing and navigating a house full of boxes. Mike was outside playing in the yard with our cat, Synlynn — a great big Siamese that our friend had rescued from the Humane Society. I looked out the window and saw Synlynn batting something around with her paws. I went outside to look just as Mike reached down to grab the object, and I yelled, "Don't pick it up!" But he was a typical 5-year-old, and he picked it up.

The object was a cotton rat — about the size of a large squirrel.

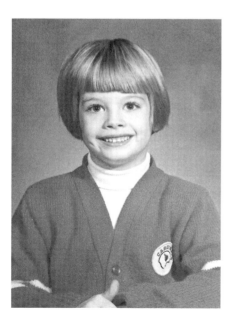

Immediately, the rat clamped its jaws down on Mike's index finger. Mike was screaming. The cotton rat was screaming. I'm sure I was screaming. Even Synlynn was screaming.

I scooped Mike up and ran in the house, but I couldn't get the rat off of his finger. My first thought was to burn a match under the rat's chin, but I was afraid I might burn Mike's finger. So instead, I set Mike and the rat on the floor and hit the rat in the jaw with a karate chop. In one fell swoop, I broke its jaw and was able to pry it open off Mike's finger.

I knew there was a possibility of rabies, so I threw the rat into one of my packing boxes, so it couldn't escape. Then I called Dr. Jim Grant — an ear, nose and throat doctor who was a great friend of ours — and told him what had happened. He said he would meet me and Mike in the Emergency Department at Le Bonheur.

I took Mike, who was bleeding, to the car and grabbed the box with the rat inside. It was a wild ride all the way down Walnut Grove Road to get to Le Bonheur. When we arrived at the ED, they immediately took Mike into a treatment room, and I handed the box to a nurse. I told her that inside was the rat that bit my son. She opened the box, saw the rat and screamed, "It's alive!" Everybody started screaming. Dr. Grant rushed out, took the box and said he would kill the rat so it could be sent off and tested for rabies.

Luckily, the rat did not have rabies, and Mike didn't even need a single stitch — just antiseptic. Mike came away from the visit relatively unscathed; I think the ED team was in worse shape than we were. It was a wild event, and I was glad to have Le Bonheur in our backyard that day.

Jorja Lynn currently resides in Holly Springs, Miss., with her husband Michael. Their son Mike lives in Cordova, Tenn., and their daughter, Lucia, lives in Holly Springs.

Little Thaxton Girl

I was born April 5, 1953, on an Easter Sunday, and I've never had another birthday on Easter since. The youngest of five children, I weighed almost 10 pounds at birth. But five weeks later, my weight had dropped to less than 7 pounds, and my parents carried me to see Dr. Theodore Rayburn in Pontotoc, Miss., near our hometown of Thaxton, Miss. Dr. Rayburn told my parents he knew something was wrong with my heart and that he was afraid I wouldn't live long; he said the best care available was at Le Bonheur Children's Hospital in Memphis, which had only been open for about six months.

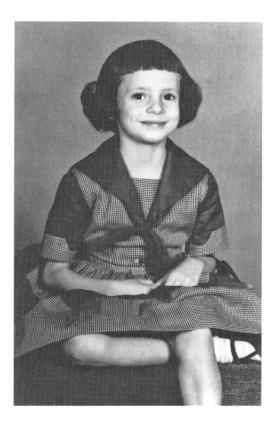

Dr. James Etteldorf was my first doctor at Le Bonheur, and he determined that I had two holes in my heart. There was no such thing as open heart surgery back in 1953, so there wasn't much they could do to fix my heart. Every week or two for the next six years, my family's old pickup made the trip up Highway 78 to Memphis, where they did EKGs and put me on a medicine called digitalis. My mother said sometimes we'd stay two weeks at a time.

Doctors told my parents that it was important to keep me from contracting childhood illnesses, so basically I sat in the house for the first six years of my life and didn't do anything except color and draw. I went to church a few times, but I could never be around other kids for fear of coming down with something. The highlight of my week was Mr. Knox Tutor, who drove the peddler truck through the countryside. Every Saturday morning, he stopped at our house and gave me a sack full of candy.

Around the time of my fifth birthday, Le Bonheur told my parents that doctors at the Mayo Clinic were developing something called open heart surgery. To be a candidate, I'd have to be at least 6 years old and weigh at least 30 pounds. When I turned 6 years old in April of 1959, I was scheduled for open heart surgery at Le Bonheur. The only thing local residents knew about the surgery was that the operation was going to cost $4,000. A fund was set up to raise money for the "little Thaxton girl that had a bad heart." Donations — usually 50 cents to a dollar — started pouring in. By the time of the surgery, more than $4,000 had been raised.

On June 25, 1959, I became the third person ever to undergo open heart surgery at Le Bonheur. Dr. Robert Allen performed the surgery along with a team of Mayo Clinic doctors, and Dr. Allen told my parents that my heart was in the worst condition of any he'd ever operated on. I was on the new heart and lung machine for more than an hour, and they used 40 pints of blood during my surgery. Following surgery, I stayed in Intensive Care for seven days. My parents weren't even allowed in the room to visit, and I remember crying because they kept it so cold in there to prevent infection.

I spent another week in the hospital in a regular room, and then my parents took me back home to Thaxton. I was young and spoiled by everyone in the county. When they gave away the car at the fair that fall, they let me draw the winning ticket. The man who won it gave me $5.

This year, I turned 59 years old. I have been married to my husband, Gary, for 41 years. We have two daughters and six grandchildren. I was born with a defective heart that couldn't be fixed and had very little chance of living, but I did live. God uses doctors and surgeries and works in all kinds of ways, and He kept me alive long enough to have the surgery I needed.

Donna Russell Pettit lives in Thaxton, Miss., with her husband, Gary. She currently works as an art teacher for North Pontotoc School.

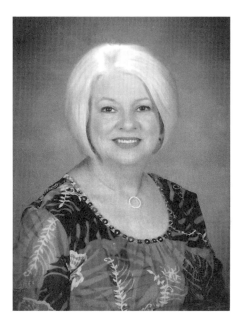

Breathing Easier

In the 1960s and 70s, it became apparent to me that Le Bonheur needed a division of pulmonary medicine to help care for and lower the death rates of infants with chronic respiratory failure, pulmonary oxygen toxicity and hyaline membrane disease. So in 1978, we established The University of Tennessee Health Science Center Division of Pulmonary Medicine.

Having a department dedicated to the treatment of patients with pulmonary issues improved their care, so that we were able to discharge children in chronic respiratory failure from Le Bonheur's Pediatric Intensive Care Unit and equip them with a home ventilator. Without a ventilator, these patients would only live for a few minutes. By having access to one at home, these babies could be with their families — a remarkable advance in patient care. Enabling these infants to live in their home environment was optimal for their normal growth and development.

Le Bonheur's Home Ventilator Program got patients out of the hospital and back at home within two or three months. Previously, this had taken two or three years. Additionally, we now had a multi-disciplinary

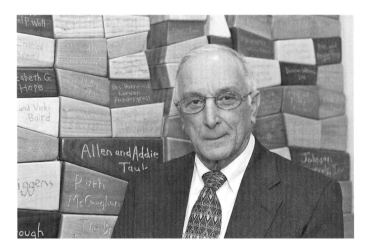

team of physicians, nurses, respiratory therapists and nutritionists who provided home care for these patients.

The Division of Pulmonary Medicine recognized a need, developed a solution and laid the foundation for those who followed to move Le Bonheur forward in pulmonary care. This was a most significant contribution to children's health care, and it leaves me with wonderful memories of where we were in 1978 and even more wonderful memories of where we are now.

Dr. Phillip George spent more than 40 years in the Department of Pediatrics at The University of Tennessee Health Science Center, during which time he served as Le Bonheur's chief of medicine, medical director of the Memphis Cystic Fibrosis Clinic and medical director of Le Bonheur's Pulmonary Function Laboratory. He is retired and lives in Memphis.

Tragedy into Triumph

My son, Brandon, was born on June 30, 1989. I had a normal pregnancy, and his was a healthy childhood. Then one afternoon when Brandon was 13, we came home from church, and he had a seizure. We went to see our pediatrician in Blytheville, Ark., and were referred to Le Bonheur.

The first time Brandon came to Le Bonheur, he stayed overnight on the old neuro unit, 5 South. At the time, I was working in Blytheville as a nurse for the state health department. Staying the night with him, I noticed that all of the nurses on the unit seemed happy and like they genuinely enjoyed their work. When they found out I was a nurse, they said I should come work here — so I did. Brandon received great, comprehensive care, and my benefits as an employee helped offset the cost of his treatment.

Brandon always wanted to help people. If you were ever sad or down, he would be the one to give you a big smile and a much-needed hug. Brandon also loved learning. He studied psychology and sociology at Arkansas Northeastern College and provided free tutoring to fellow students — even though his school offered financial compensation to student tutors. He gave rides to single parents without transportation, so that they could consistently attend class. In 2009, he gave a presentation to the Rockefeller Foundation and helped his college obtain a grant to provide financial resources for single parents, individuals with disabilities or students involved in community service. He was a mentor and a source of inspiration for many of his peers.

In August of 2009, Brandon died from sudden unexpected epilepsy death — a condition in which a healthy individual with epilepsy passes away abruptly, without an apparent cause. When Brandon died, his school established the Brandon J. Elliott Memorial Scholarship to continue his legacy of helping others. Since his death, we have awarded seven scholarships to individuals in need of assistance. My husband and I don't want to let our sadness cause us not to help somebody else. We have decided to turn tragedy into triumph.

Each year, I participate in a walk for the Epilepsy Foundation of Florida in West Palm Beach, Fla., where Brandon was born. Brandon's son, Brandon, Jr. — who was born two months after his father's passing — attends the event with us in memory of his daddy.

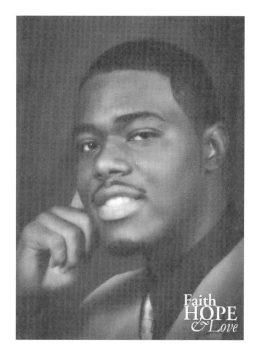

I think that Le Bonheur is a special place. There are many places where nurses can work, but it's not often that you find a place with such care and compassion for the human element — where your job is more than just a paycheck and a means to support your family. While it was my son who brought me here, I stay because of the people here who believe so strongly in what we do.

Cassandra Elliott has served as a nurse on Le Bonheur's Flex team for seven years. She and her husband, Jerome, reside in Blytheville.

Poochie

I came to Le Bonheur as a pediatric resident in 1962. Back in the 60s, if you were at the hospital but weren't really on call, you could pass the time sunbathing up on the roof. I've joked around that the house officers — residents — used to drink beer on the roof and throw the cans at passing cars. But of course, that's not really true. What is true, though, is that there was a conference room on the fourth floor of the hospital with a beautiful leather couch. The house officers went up there so often to make out that the administrators started locking the door and closed off the room.

I often flirted with the nurses, and I remember one beautiful nurse named June who caught my eye. I asked one of the fellow residents, Bob Stewart, to introduce me to June because he had already worked with her. He said alright, and then told me she was expecting me to meet her at a certain place and time in town. On the big day, I went to meet this lady and introduced myself, saying, "Bob Stewart told me to meet you here. He said he was a good friend of yours." She looked up and said, "Who the hell is Bob Stewart?" He'd set me up, and I was so embarrassed, but June and I turned out to be good friends.

Back then, we had quite a few chronic patients who were ambulatory, and to help keep them occupied and moving, sometimes we would include them on rounds. I remember one child named Poochie who had nephrosis. Every time we made our rounds, we put Poochie in a white coat, and he would make rounds, too. We'd always ask him his opinion, and he'd say things like, "Well, I agree with that diagnosis."

One of my greatest moments was during a financial crisis in

the 1970s. The administrators and key physicians were having a big meeting in the board room, and everyone was pouring over the charts and numbers. I borrowed a huge Afro wig from one of my technicians, eased on in to the conference room and sat down. Everyone saw me and started laughing, and they relaxed after that.

We once treated a patient who was the son of one of the pediatricians. The child had developed congenital herpes, and he had blisters all over his scalp after he was born. We really had no idea what to do for a newborn with herpes. Worried that the child would suffer brain damage, we broke all the blisters on his head, and I bathed his head in any type of antiviral medicine I

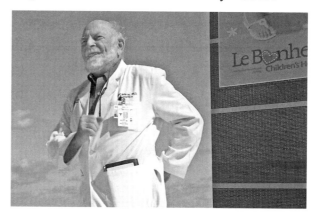

could find. Eventually the child made a full recovery. Last I heard, he graduated from college and was a first-string football player. It was a great success story for us at that time.

I've been at Le Bonheur for 50 years and treated many children who have come through the doors here. I'm glad that Le Bonheur can serve as home for these children when they need us. 🤍

Dr. Sid Wilroy has worked at Le Bonheur Children's Hospital for 50 years. He lives in Memphis with his wife, Lynn.

Behind the Scenes

I work in the Facilities Services department at Le Bonheur now, but my first experience at the hospital was as a mother. My son, Blake, had surgery at Le Bonheur in 1994, when he was only 4 months old.

When Blake was 2 months old, I noticed that his head wasn't taking a normal shape. A bony ridge was starting to develop in the center of his forehead. We were living in our hometown of Florence, Ala., at the time. I asked his doctor about it, and he dismissed it at first, but then on the next visit he diagnosed Blake with metopic synostosis, which meant the sutures in his skull had fused prematurely. He needed surgery to repair his facial deformity.

Two months later, we arrived at Le Bonheur for his surgery. I stayed with Blake in his room most of time while he recovered from his operation, but eventually we ventured out to explore the hospital. The lobby was new, and we loved that there was so much for the kids to do. My niece and older son, Brandon, loved the train, the lights that twirled, the blinking stars and animal sounds.

Blake recovered well after surgery, but we knew we'd have to come back for monthly visits with his surgeon, Dr. Michael Muhlbauer.

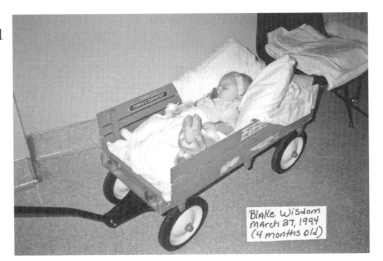

Blake Wisdom
March 27, 1994
(4 months old)

My first thought was, "My goodness, how are we going to afford that?" We had a newspaper with us and happened upon a help-wanted ad for a Memphis position with my husband's company. While we were in Blake's hospital room, we started thinking about moving to Memphis because we would have to come back so often.

My husband applied and interviewed for the position, and we've been in Memphis ever since. It's Le Bonheur that brought us here. In 2010, I quit a job I didn't enjoy and applied to work at Le Bonheur. My first day was June 1 — two weeks before the hospital's grand opening ceremony. It was weird to walk through the same lobby I'd brought my son through in 1994. This time, the new hospital was being constructed, and renovations on the existing lobby were beginning. I still had a brand new ceiling and walls with neon lights pictured in my mind, but everything was outdated and being torn down.

Walking through the new hospital, it's nice to see the same child-friendly elements incorporated throughout, just as they were before. It's awesome being part of the Le Bonheur team. What we do, the families may not always see. But it's what we do behind the scenes that impacts them and makes their stay better. I knew that then as a mom, and I still know and believe that now.

Nancy Wisdom is the O&M Operations supervisor at Le Bonheur. She and her husband, Terry, live in Hernando, Miss., with their son, Blake, who graduated high school this year and wants to be an architect. Their older son, Brandon, lives in Jonesboro, Ark.

Like Magic

I came to Le Bonheur in 2002 as the newest member of Pediatric Surgery Group. I joined the team so that Dr. Robert Hollabaugh could retire. Dr. Hollabaugh was a legend, and while I was glad to be on the team, I was disappointed that I wouldn't have an opportunity to work with him. However, about six months after I came on board, Dr. Hollabaugh came out of retirement for awhile to help out while another partner was ill.

Working with him was such a blessing. Dr. Hollabaugh had such a high standard and had seen everything, while I was newly out of fellowship and was still learning. Often in those early years, I would see conditions with which I was unfamiliar, so I would call Dr. Hollabaugh for advice. His reply to me was always, "Trey, I see something new every day." Coming from such a brilliant surgeon, this response was very encouraging to me.

One trauma stands out in my memory of my early days at Le Bonheur. A patient came in who was critically injured — an unsurvivable injury — but we wanted to operate to see if there was anything we could do to save this child. At that time, nights and weekends weren't heavily staffed in the Operating Room, and when I began surgery, our team included only an anesthesiologist, a pediatric surgery fellow, a nurse, a scrub tech and a CRNA. I put my head down and began to work on repairing this child.

We worked for hours. Every time I asked for something — an instrument, more blood, anything — it appeared like magic, so that I could keep working. Eventually, despite our efforts, the child died. When I looked up, eyes filled with tears, I noticed that the room and hallway was filled with people who had returned to help with the surgery. Nurses, techs and others came in from home and from other units on a weekend night to do everything they could to save this child. That's when I knew Le Bonheur was the right place for me to work. This hospital isn't bricks and mortar; it's people who have developed a culture based on love and sacrifice for the kids we care for every day.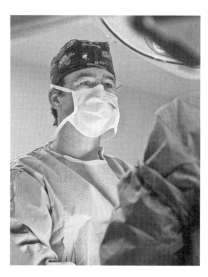

Dr. James Wallace "Trey" Eubanks, III, is a general surgeon with Pediatric Surgery Group and serves as the medical director of Trauma Services for Le Bonheur Children's Hospital. He currently lives in Memphis with his wife, Angela, and their children.

My Dream

The Creative Arts room at Le Bonheur opened not long after I started working here. My department, Child Life, often used the room to host arts and crafts activities for patients. The activities weren't really meant to be a profound experience; they were simply intended as a fun way to pass the time and help keep our patients entertained.

One afternoon, we invited children to come by the Creative Arts room and make mobiles. The activity theme was dreams for the future. A number of patients participated in the project, including a 10-year-old boy who had cystic fibrosis. This child was a frequent flyer at Le Bonheur. He was probably admitted to the hospital four or five times a year, and typically he stayed for two or three weeks at a time. He really grew up at Le Bonheur, and everybody knew him.

He was a very happy-go-lucky child — the kind of kid you see walking around the hospital, always smiling.

In the Creative Arts room that day, everyone approached their mobiles differently. Some children cut out pictures and created a collage of images. Others drew pictures or decorated their designs with stickers. Many wrote phrases such as "I want to be a football player," and "I dream of

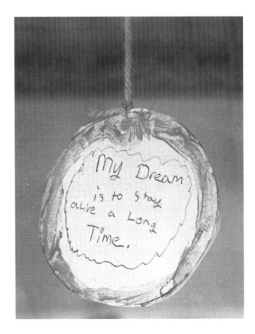

becoming a movie star." Our frequent flyer stopped by to participate and left his mobile on a table with the others. It wasn't until we were cleaning up the activity that we saw he had written, "My dream is to stay alive a long time."

This child was always happy, upbeat and comfortable in his surroundings. None of us had any clue that, internally, he was struggling with his own mortality. When we saw his project, we were able to speak with his treatment team and make them aware of his concerns. The mobile started a dialogue between us and the patient that continued throughout the course of his hospitalization.

This was an unforgettable moment that illustrated the importance of each of our interactions with these kids. We were able to create an environment where, for a moment in time, this child felt safe enough to tell us what he was thinking. His mobile hung in the Creative Arts room for years as a reminder of the importance of the work we do and of the impact all of us can have on a life.

Thomas Hobson has worked at Le Bonheur Children's for 10 years and currently serves as the director of Child Life. He lives in Memphis with his wife, Becky, and their children, Andrew and Lauren.

Dr. E.

My father, Dr. James N. Etteldorf, was affectionately known around the halls of The University of Tennessee Health Science Center as Dr. E. He was one of the champions of the drive to build a children's hospital during the early 1940s. Later, Dad served as Le Bonheur's chief of staff from 1961-65.

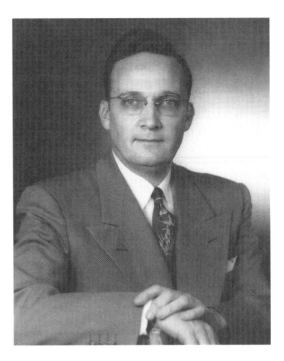

When I was a little girl, I had an appendectomy. There was no bed for me in any children's facility, so I had to stay in the maternity ward at John Gaston Hospital. I was so embarrassed.

When the Le Bonheur Club ladies came to my father to help plan a children's hospital for Memphis, Dad was one of their biggest champions. He knew there were not enough hospital beds for children in the city, so Daddy led the push to advocate for the construction of a pediatric hospital.

My father was interested in medicine from an early age. As a teenager in the 1920s, he would travel with the local doctor by horse and wagon to visit patients on the Sioux Indian reservation near his home town of Lenox, S.D. It was then that he developed a love for healing and decided to become a doctor.

Dad was a compassionate man, and he used to say there was no such word as "can't." When patients couldn't afford to go to the hospital, he went out of his way to help them. Once, a patient who didn't have much money paid my father in strawberries, which he happily accepted. I remember another patient named Jeff who had nephritis — inflammation of the kidneys — and at that time, there was no cure for his illness. Jeff's family was unable to pay $35 a day for a hospital room, so Dad and I would go to his home, and Dad would perform the necessary treatments for his illness. I would assist my dad by handing him syringes and other instruments, and when Jeff died, he left a note saying he wanted me — "Dr. Jim's girl"— to have his horse, Lady.

Dad is recognized for contributing many firsts to Memphis pediatrics, including the use of penicillin in treating meningitis, ACTH for the treatment of leukemia and nephrosis and the successful treatment of tuberculosis meningitis. He practiced pediatric nephrology before it was a subspecialty, and he was the first to perform peritoneal dialysis on a child in Memphis. My father's colleagues called him "the father of academic pediatrics in Memphis" for his contributions to medical education, pediatric care and clinical research.

My father's purpose in life was to make a difference, and had he not been such an idealist and pushed so hard, Le Bonheur may never have been. I know he would be so excited and proud if he could see the new hospital today.

Dr. James Etteldorf died in 1997 at the age of 87. His daughter, Eleanor Etteldorf Nunn, lives with her husband, Warren, in Halls, Tenn. Eleanor and Warren, Eleanor's sister — Marcella Houseal of Memphis — and their children and grandchildren celebrated Dr. Etteldorf's legacy at the grand opening of the new Le Bonheur on June 15, 2010. The couple named a room in the new hospital in memory of Dr. and Mrs. James Nickolas Etteldorf.

The Way It Was

I worked at Le Bonheur for 31 years, but my most vivid memory is when my son, David, was a patient there. In January of 1989, my son was born after a 50-hour labor. We knew he would be born with a birth defect that required immediate attention, so we planned to have him transferred to Le Bonheur when he was just a few hours old. Dr. Hollabaugh performed surgery on him, and then my son spent two days in the Pediatric Intensive Care Unit followed by two weeks on 7 Central, the surgery floor.

After two weeks of excellent care we transferred to 5 South — the hospital's newest unit. It was lovely being in a brand new room on a brand new unit. All of the staff were wonderful, making sure I was comfortable after such a long delivery and providing tender care for my premature infant. I received all of my meals because I was a nursing mother, which was extremely convenient because I could not easily leave my newborn to go get food for myself. Despite the scary situation, we were supported in every way throughout my son's recovery, and I will never forget the manner in which the Le Bonheur staff cared for us.

Shortly after I returned to work, another baby boy was admitted who was very close to David in age. This patient was admitted frequently as he was ill with a chronic condition, and I often provided care for him as his dietitian. The baby's mother and I developed a close bond because our sons were almost the same age. At times, I felt that I was caring for my own son. Although I was sorry when the patient had to be admitted, I was always happy to see the family and help them in any way that I could. That's the way it was for me over the years. Bonding with our families always enriched my time working at Le Bonheur. My time there will always hold a special place in my heart.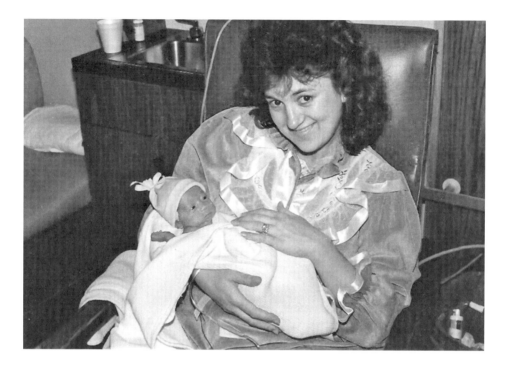

Ginger Carney served as a Le Bonheur staff member from 1978-2009. Most recently, she held the role of director of Clinical Nutrition. Her son, David, is an aerospace/ocean engineering major at Virginia Tech.

Birthday Bag

When I was 19 weeks pregnant, I went for an ultrasound to find out if I was having a boy or a girl; I suspected I was having a girl. The ultrasound detected gastroschisis — a condition in which a baby's intestines stick out of the body through a defect in the umbilical cord — and hydrocephalus, a buildup of fluid inside the skull that can cause brain swelling. I was referred to a maternal-fetal medicine specialist who confirmed the diagnoses, and I began interviewing doctors at Le Bonheur and touring the hospital's Neonatal Intensive Care and Special Care Units.

At 37 weeks, Emma made her debut. She was born at Methodist Germantown and taken via Pedi-Flite helicopter to Le Bonheur when she was only 2 hours old. Her first surgery was performed when she was 4 hours old. The doctors returned Emma's intestines to her abdomen and made her the most adorable little belly button. Today, you would never know that she was born with her "insides on the outside."

Eight days later, Emma underwent her second surgery at Le Bonheur — the placement of a shunt in her brain. She spent a total of 40 days at Le Bonheur before I finally took her home.

Emma and I were back at Le Bonheur a number of times during that first year. Two weeks shy of her first birthday, Emma had a seizure while sitting in her car seat. I frantically called 911 and begged the ambulance to take us to Le Bonheur, even though it was not the closest hospital. It took us a while to figure out her seizure triggers and get the daily medicines right, and Emma spent June and July of 2008 in and out of the Emergency Department with seizures.

On the day of her first birthday party in June 2008, Emma had a seizure that sent us to the ED. That was the day I first really felt the power of Child Life. One of the ED nurses told Child Life that Emma was missing her first birthday party. Soon, Child Life arrived with a birthday bag for Emma — a pink cloth

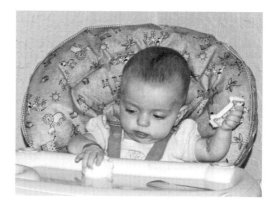

bag with a small purple Mylar balloon, a Puffalump stuffed toy and an age-appropriate soft teething book about farm animals on a ring. We kept the balloon for nearly two years, and the book was attached to her stroller for a long time.

We made it home that night in time to celebrate Emma's birthday a little late but surrounded by friends. Pictures from that day show Emma smiling, still a bit groggy, wearing Band-Aids on her arms. Emma's first birthday was not our last visit to Le Bonheur, but the memory of the nurses and Child Life working in concert to bring a little joy to a stressful moment has not faded.

Jessica Huntley serves on Le Bonheur's Family Partners Council and is chair of the council's Staff Education Committee. She and Emma reside in Memphis. Emma is 5 years old.

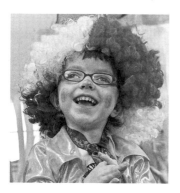

One Big Family

I came to Le Bonheur in 1974, and my first job was working as a unit secretary on the surgery floor. Back then, surgery was located on the first floor of the hospital, and the building only went up four stories. The hospital was much more intimate then; you knew everybody. We grew really close with many of the parents, and some of them would come over to my house for visits. There were even times when I would take patients home to spend the night on the weekends if they didn't have family around. The whole hospital was one big family.

I've seen many firsts and a great deal of change in my time at Le Bonheur. I remember working on the surgery floor when we did our first heart transplant. The building that is now Le Bonheur's Research Center used to be a patio with swings and a little playground for the kids. That's where the West Tower went up. We had a gift shop and drug store right off the main entrance at 848 Adams St., and inside there was a little snack bar. Another part of our campus, the Education and Support Centers, used to be a Chevrolet car lot. I've watched Le Bonheur grow up around me.

When the surgery unit moved from the first floor up to the seventh floor, I remember how pretty it was for us. Our old unit was in one of the original parts of the building, and we still had iron beds for the patients. When we moved up to the new part, we really felt like we were going somewhere. We'd never been up that high before — none of us had — and they had fish tanks in the playrooms with live fish swimming around.

Sometimes celebrities visited the hospital, and that was always something fun to do with the kids. I remember once there was a

burn patient on my unit, and she loved to be out at the nurses'
station with me. Blues singer Ruby Wilson came to visit, and this
child and I had our picture made with her. Another time, Willie
Stargell — a baseball player for the Pittsburgh Pirates — visited
Le Bonheur, and I had my picture made with him.

Le Bonheur has been my life, and I have always — I'll say it over
and over again — loved it because of the kids. Holding babies at the
nurses' station, comforting the children when their parents were not
here — those are the fondest memories for me. 💙

*Countess Hearn has worked at Le Bonheur since 1974. She has worked as a unit
secretary and currently serves as a scheduler on the Patient Access team.*

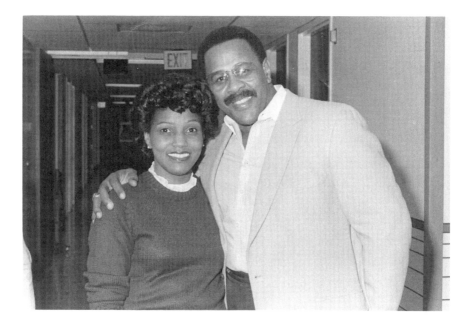

Joining Forces

In the spring of 1995, I received a phone call from Gene Cashman, the CEO of Le Bonheur Children's. At the time, I was serving as chief operating officer of Methodist Healthcare, and Gene called to ask if Methodist might be interested in bringing our two organizations together. While we weren't sure how that might take shape — as a purchase, merger or other transaction — one of the more exciting moments in my career was the opportunity to sit down and explore this possibility with Gene. Even in the mid-90s, Le Bonheur had such a strong regional presence, and we knew if Methodist could work out an alignment agreement, it would really strengthen the position of the whole health system.

Initially, Le Bonheur was interested in developing a community model with Baptist and Methodist, in which the two multi-hospital systems and Le Bonheur would share pediatric care in the community. When that idea didn't take root, Le Bonheur decided to explore a joint venture with one system. While Gene was certainly interested in the financial stability and growth opportunity for Le Bonheur, what impressed me most was his vested interest in improving the health status for women and children in Memphis and the surrounding areas.

In July of that year, Gene and I drafted a document about a women and children's center of excellence, rooted in community outreach and community focus. From that document grew LHS — Le Bonheur Health Systems, Inc. — a foundation focused on the well-being and health of children in our community. Today, LHS is known in Memphis as The Urban Child Institute, and Gene Cashman serves at the helm.

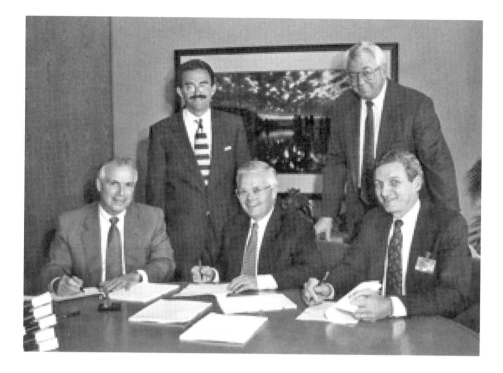

In October of 1995, Methodist Health Systems and Le Bonheur Children's Medical Center joined forces to become Methodist Le Bonheur Healthcare. At the first board meeting following the alignment, I invited Le Bonheur's hospital puppet to come and meet with the board. This was well received, and people had a good time with it. For me, that cemented the idea that we had become a different organization. Our focus would include children from then on; it was fun.

The merger allowed Methodist to improve Le Bonheur's financial position while strengthening our own presence in the community. Despite the obvious initial benefits, I don't think Gene or I could have envisioned Le Bonheur as it exists today — a beacon of hope and healing on the corner of Poplar and Dunlap. It has far exceeded anything we expected to see.

I think the most important asset any community has is children, and how those children are cared for is an indication of the overall health of the community. I couldn't be more proud of what Le Bonheur does for kids from every quadrant of our city. Our children have access to the same physicians, the same nurses and the same technology. To me, that is a source of great pride — not just for us at Methodist Le Bonheur, but for our entire community.

Gary Shorb joined Methodist in 1990. Since 2001, he has served as president and CEO of Methodist Healthcare. In addition to his work at Methodist, Gary serves on the boards of Memphis Tomorrow, the National Civil Rights Museum, the Memphis Regional Chamber of Commerce, the Memphis Bioworks Foundation and the University of Memphis Board of Visitors.

I'll Take Care of Her

My daughter, Ava, was born in 2007. When she was just an infant, my husband and I brought her to Le Bonheur. She breathed like she was running a race, and she would sweat while she ate. Doctors diagnosed Ava with VSD — a congenital heart defect — and kidney reflux. She had surgery when she was only 3 months old and stayed at Le Bonheur for a month, so she could heal.

I remember going to see Ava after open heart surgery. She had tubes and machines hooked up to her tiny body, helping her breathe. Soon, they moved us to the Special Care Unit. I was so tired. Ava was eating every two hours, and between the lack of sleep and the stress of her being in the hospital, I was so exhausted I could barely manage.

One night, Ava started crying because she wanted to eat. I started to get up and feed her. A nurse came in and said, "You sleep. I'll feed Ava. You need your rest. I'll take care of her." This simple gesture meant the absolute world to me. It meant that this nurse — all of the nurses — understood my needs, as well as Ava's. The entire staff at Le Bonheur saw the needs of my whole family and took care of us. You don't get that at other hospitals.

After Ava was released from the hospital, she was on several different medications for a long time. Giving medicine to a baby every day is a real challenge. One day, we went for a follow-up clinic appointment. At the end of our visit, Dr. Chin said that Ava didn't have to take medicine anymore. I stopped, looked hard at him and said, "Excuse me? Say that again?" He started laughing and repeated it. I just couldn't believe it and was so relieved. No more medicine!

To see your child so vulnerable and sick is something no mom ever wants to see. But Le Bonheur gives the gift of life. The doctors there had the skill and expertise to diagnose and treat all of Ava's conditions, and they fixed her heart. Because of Le Bonheur, I have my Ava.

Allison Fuché and her husband live in Memphis with their three children. Ava is 5 years old.

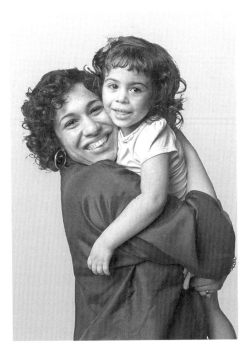

Making the Cut

I n the early 1980s,
Le Bonheur thought of
itself as a regional center — a
hospital serving Memphis
and the area 100 miles
around. When we came here
in 1985 to start the Brain
Tumor Program at St. Jude
and Le Bonheur, no one
believed in the importance of
surgery in cancer treatment.
Treatment relied on radiation
and chemotherapy. As we

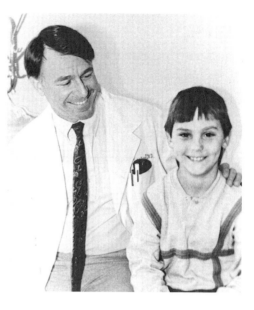

began to build up the program, I met with Le Bonheur's CEO and
asked him if he would fully support us on the surgical side, as well as
accept any and all patients in need. He said yes — we'd proceed for a
year, and at the end of the year, if we broke even or better, we'd do it
again the next year. With a handshake, we changed the scope of care
for children with brain tumors. Our arrangement also ensured that
all a child had to do to be accepted to our program was show up at
the front door.

One of my favorite stories from those days is about a child from
Louisiana. This patient was diagnosed with a brain tumor, and his
family had no money, so they were sent to a hospital in Louisiana
that was not equipped to care for his condition. Next they went to
Texas Children's in Houston, but they were deferred for treatment
because they were not Texas residents. Somehow they found out that

they could come to Le Bonheur and receive care, so they drove to Memphis. On the way, their car broke down, and they hitchhiked with their child all the way to the front doors of Le Bonheur. We performed surgery on the child. He did very well and is still living today. We've had similar referrals many times, and we've never turned anyone away.

Another patient who stands out is a young girl whose family had been told at two other top hospitals that their child's brain tumor was inoperable. They went online and found our program. When I met with them, I told them I could successfully remove her tumor, and I did. The child went to the Pediatric Intensive Care Unit after her surgery, but she was feeling so well and crawling out of bed that we moved her up to the neuro unit that same day. The next morning, Tracy Tidwell and I were rounding together. When we walked in the room, the little girl was standing with her nose in the corner. I asked what was going on, and the child's mother said, "She hit her father, and she's in time out." I just laughed and said, "If a child's well enough to get in time out, she's well enough to go home." So we sent her home, and she's still doing great to this day.

Since 1985, our program has found that with the three most common types of brain tumors in children, you double the cure rate if you surgically remove the entire tumor before starting chemo and radiation. We've progressed from a 30 percent cure rate to an 80 percent cure rate for these patients and have proven the importance of surgery. Throughout 27 years here, my experience has been that Le Bonheur is people — physicians, nurses, therapists and others who are dedicated to what's best for kids. So often, we work against very long odds. It's people who make the difference.

Dr. Robert A. Sanford joined Semmes-Murphey Clinic in 1985 and founded the Brain Tumor Program at Le Bonheur Children's and St. Jude Children's Research Hospital.

Dog Day

I am crazy about the George Rodrigue Blue Dog painting that hangs on Le Bonheur's first floor. Located in the hospital's Hall of Mirrors, I would often detour down the hallway on my way to the chapel, just so I could greet the grinning blue canine aloud. When I passed the painting, I greeted him just like I do my own dog, Abby. "How'z ya do-zing? Having a good dog day?"

Since Blue Dog has arrived at Le Bonheur, I discovered him to be a perfect distraction for comforting young, scared patients. There's just something about the power of the Blue Dog. One day, just after I'd said my morning greeting to big Blue, I heard a shriek and turned to see a little fellow about 6 years old racing toward me. We nearly collided in his apparent attempt to escape a clinic appointment; his mother was hot on his heels.

The little boy stopped short, looking at me to determine whether I was friend or foe. As our eyes met, I asked him, "Have you ever seen a blue dog?" He paused, then told me there was no such thing. "Yes there is," I responded. "I'll show him to you."

I held his little fingers in my hand and led him to the painting. He looked up, pointed excitedly and shouted, "A blue dog!" He was smiling for the first time since I'd seen him. But after thinking a moment, he said, "It's not a real dog."

"Speak to him," I said. The boy looked up at me, puzzled.

"I usually say, 'Blue Dog, how'z ya do-zing? Having a good dog day?' Go ahead. Try it. Speak to him."

The child hesitated and weighed his options — make a break for it or talk to the dog. Then he leaned in close to Blue's right foreleg and planted a kiss. He whispered, "Hey, Blue Dog."

By that time, he was grinning and laughing as his mother took his hand and led him peacefully back to the clinic. I figure a place that has a giant blue dog can't be all that bad. That's his power. Time just stops when kids see him. 🩷

Ann Phillips is a board-certified pediatric chaplain and an ordained UCC minister. She worked as a chaplain at Le Bonheur until 2011 and currently serves as a chaplain for acute liver failure and home hospice patients.

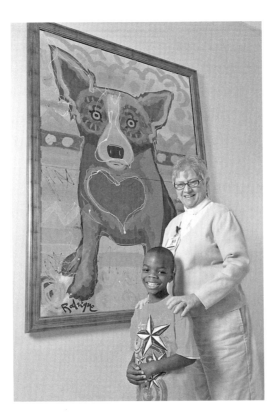

Gold Tags

I joined Le Bonheur Club in 1964, and Sue Cheek Hughes was my new member leader at the time. Sue and her father, Memphis architect J. Frazer Smith, actually designed the original Le Bonheur Children's Hospital. Sue was a good leader, and she trained us well.

When I got in the club, I was seven months pregnant. We were selling gold tags — bumper stickers in support of Le Bonheur — for $10, and the minimum you had to raise was $200. I was new to town and didn't know anyone, but my husband gave me the names of some family friends, and I went around town selling my gold tags. Everyone bought tags from me because I was a pregnant woman asking for money.

We also sold something called March tags, which were bumper stickers that corresponded with license tag renewals. Back then, all

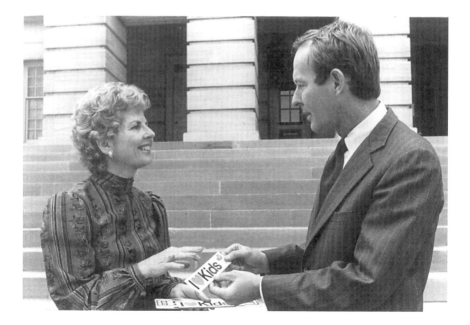

license tags were sold during March, and we would sell March tags for 50 cents at the fairgrounds, the courthouse and anywhere else they were selling license tags. We would work in shifts of four or five for three hours, and we made quite a bit of money — sometimes $20,000 in a month. It was very busy; you were on your feet the whole time. We had the gold tags available there, too, but hardly anyone ever had that much money.

Selling tags was a wonderful experience because people would come up and give you all the change in their pocket, and then they would tell stories about their children or nieces or grandchildren who had been at Le Bonheur. We heard lots of stories and told stories of our own, and as club members, we got to know one another really well. At times we felt guilty because we knew people didn't really have the money to give, but they thought so much of the hospital that they wanted to give it anyway.

Eventually gold tags went from $10 to $25. We sold many of these tags to business men in the community, and we went to their offices to call on them. There was no e-mail, and you didn't do it by phone — that just wasn't done — so you got dressed up in heels and a nice dress, and you went out and called on these offices. And if you had all day, you did it all day. Pat Klinke was the queen of these calls because she made a rum cake for every person she called on. She even sold a tag once to Tennessee Gov. Lamar Alexander.

As the years went on, people donated wonderful prizes that we could win depending on how much money we raised selling gold tags. The contests were always fun, but we did the work because we loved helping the children. Le Bonheur was our happiness.

Billie Anne Williams has been a Le Bonheur Club member for 48 years. She served as club president in 1976 and has also served on the board of Le Bonheur Children's Hospital. Club members Gloria Andereck and Elaine Colmer contributed memories to this story.

I'll Carry Him Now

I gave birth to my third child, Jay, in the summer of 1985. My husband, Hamp, and I were excited about having another baby. It had been a normal pregnancy, and it seemed like a normal delivery.

I still remember the minute he was born, a hush came over the delivery room. The doctor came back to the table to finish with me, and he said, "You have a little boy, but he was born with a hole in his cord," My first thoughts were, "That's his umbilical cord; we don't need that anymore." Then the doctor said the hole was in his spinal cord and I thought, "Lord, don't do this to me."

Jay's diagnosis was spina bifida. The neurosurgeon told us that he would probably be mentally retarded, never walk and be paralyzed from his chest down. We were in a fog; we felt like this was not really happening. The first few weeks were tough, but then we started to settle in. We knew we were going to have a child who was paralyzed from the chest down, and we were going to press on.

When Jay was a baby, I remember thinking that I would do anything for Le Bonheur. It was an amazing thing to go from having never needed Le Bonheur to being there every day — day and night. Hamp and I walked the halls of that hospital many a night, late at night, wondering how things were going to turn out the next day. That's when you meet some special people. You meet a nurse who's doing her books and writing in her logs. You go have a cup of coffee with someone, you talk to a janitor who is polishing floors, and you know that everybody loves the kids. Le Bonheur is the people who work there — from the doctors and nurses to the people in the cafeteria and the people working the desks on the floors.

Our son underwent 28 surgeries at Le Bonheur during his lifetime; 21 of them were major. He loved company. People would call to check on him, and he'd say, "Come see me!" He was a gatherer of people, and he had an incredible ability to relate to those around him. Jay's ability to rejoice in his friend's abilities was unbelievable, and it drew people to him.

If children with spina bifida live past age 4, they usually live into adulthood. We expected for Jay to live. But for some particular reason, that was not what the Lord had planned.

On June 15, 1999 — just a regular day, with a house full of out-of-town company — I went up to get Jay, and the Lord had taken him home in the night. It was three days before his 14th birthday.

We took Jay down to our bedroom, dressed him and laid him on the bed. Within 30 minutes, 50 people were in our home. We sang "Amazing Grace" around his bed and prayed, and everyone shared the effects that Jay had on their lives. Children in the neighborhood were able to come kiss him and touch him and say goodbye.

After about two hours, an ambulance came to take Jay to the funeral home. We were both ready. They asked us if we needed a stretcher, and 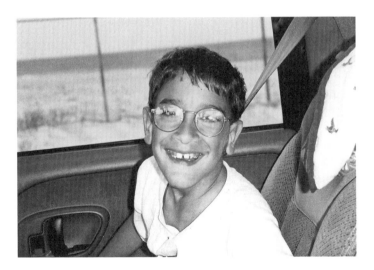 Hamp said, "No. I've carried him all his life. I'll carry him now."

So he carried him out, and we followed. Hamp laid Jay on the stretcher. We turned around and looked, and the walkway up to our house was lined with our friends and our family. Every window was covered with faces, and every eye was filled with tears. It was sad, but there was such a spirit that this boy is free — and he's walking, and he's talking, and he's praising his King.

First Corinthians 4:1 says, "Let a man regard us as stewards of the mysteries of God." I think the way God used Jay's life was to touch people. Everybody's hurting. Everybody feels paralyzed in some form or another, and it's just as painful as if you are physically paralyzed. When people saw Jay living with joy and acceptance of what God had given him — a true surrender of the soul — then they were able to think, "There is hope."

Hamp and Nancy Holcomb currently reside in Memphis and continue to advocate for and support Le Bonheur.